Case Studies
in
Cultural Diversity

Case Studies
in
Cultural Diversity

A WORKBOOK

Vernice D. Ferguson, Editor

JONES AND BARTLETT PUBLISHERS
Sudbury, Massachusetts
BOSTON   TORONTO   LONDON   SINGAPORE

World Headquarters
Jones and Bartlett Publishers
40 Tall Pine Drive
Sudbury, MA 01776
978-443-5000

info@jbpub.com
www.jbpub.com

Jones and Bartlett Publishers International
Barb House, Barb Mews
London W6 7PA
UK

Jones and Bartlett Publishers Canada
P.O. Box 19020
Toronto, ON M5S 1X1
CANADA

Copyright © 1999 by Jones and Bartlett Publishers, Inc.

The views expressed in this publication represent the views of the authors and do not necessarily reflect the official views of the National League for Nursing.

Library of Congress Cataloging-in-Publication Data

Case studies in cultural diversity : a workbook / Vernice D.
Ferguson, editor.
    p. cm. — (Pub.)
    Includes bibliographical references and index.
    ISBN 0-7637-0921-2
    1. Transcultural nursing. 2. Transcultural nursing—Case
studies. I. Ferguson, Vernice. II. Series: Pub. (National League
for Nursing)
    [DNLM: 1. Community Health Nursing. 2. Cultural Diversity. WY
106 C337 1998]
RT86.54.C37   1998
610.73—ddc21

                  97–46651
                  CIP

Printed in the United States of America
02 01 00 99 98 10 9 8 7 6 5 4 3 2 1

CONTENTS

Contents

Page 3   Vernice Ferguson teaching a science class at a local high school. Washington, D.C.

Page 19   Nurse in the village clinic demonstrating procedure to nursing student.

Page 29   Inner city healthcare involves all family members.

Page 47   A CHN student measuring child's arm circumference for malnutrition screening.

Page 59   Southern Illinois University at Edwardsville, School of Nursing, Community Nursing Services.

Page 75   This Bolivian woman had buried a son the previous day, a victim of whooping cough. The visiting nurse offered advice on how to avoid further tragedies in her family.

Page 85   For the old people confronted with disease, the visiting nurse is part of the family.

Page 99   Examination of a pregnant woman by Kulwinder Kaur.

Page 107   Weighing a new-born baby. Training in South-East Asia reflects the new approaches to rural healthcare.

Page 121   Nurse in the village clinic demonstrating procedure to nursing student.

Page 131   Interview of a patient in the home setting is an important opportunity to establish rapport.

Page 139   For the aged, the nurse is "one of the family."

Page 149   Homecare nursing is an important part of the University of Pennsylvania program.

Page 165   Kulwinder Kaur teaches health to young students.

Page 179   Cultural values must be accepted and integrated into nursing care. This family is from Mozambique.

Page 191   Touching is an important part of caring in home healthcare.

Page 197   Giving shots and practicing vaccination are part of the training of the ENI students.

PREFACE

*T*his book of case studies is an outgrowth of a grant received from the Independence Foundation, a privately funded foundation located in Philadelphia, Pennsylvania. The foundation has funded chairs for nurse scholars in a number of schools of nursing. In addition, grants have been provided to nurse investigators who seek to improve nursing education. The Foundation has shown particular interest in collaborative activities among schools of nursing.

This grant, "Preparing Nurses for America's Multicultural Future," provided the opportunity for faculty from schools of nursing in the Delaware Valley area to work together to develop case studies that are community-focused and culturally sensitive. Represented in this collection are case studies developed by nursing faculty members at Gwynedd-Mercy College, Jefferson, LaSalle, Temple, Villanova, the University of Pennsylvania, and Widener University. This approach should prove useful as we prepare nursing students to respond to the new realities in healthcare.

The case studies are planned for use with baccalaureate nursing students. Community-focused care is coming into its own in a nation that has relied heavily on hospitals as the major site for delivering healthcare services. In the past, schools of nursing used the lecture method almost exclusively to teach students. With the shift to providing more care in the community, the case study method becomes a more useful approach.

Faculty members require guidance as well, for there is new knowledge to be acquired and attitudes adjusted as we move in this challenging new direction. As we developed the case studies, we considered some essential values and behaviors that characterize college and university education for professional nursing. We kept in mind the final report of the American Association of Colleges of Nursing, *Essentials of College and University Education for Nursing* (1986). Our goals became an opportunity to:

1. Develop an awareness of the impact of culture in the provision of nursing care.
2. Enhance the healthcare of people through improved relationships between healthcare providers and their recipients.
3. Facilitate improved care in a multicultural environment through the empowerment of the recipients of nursing services.
4. Increase the knowledge base of teacher and student through the use of case studies that consider the impact of culture and the community on care provision.

During the course of the collaborative faculty initiative to develop these case studies, I was privileged to have spent nine weeks in South Africa among nurses, nursing students, and those served by them. From tertiary hospitals and their clinics in large cities to townships and village hospitals and clinics, nursing homes, hospices, squatter camps and homes of the people, nursing's work to improve health and support the hopelessly ill was readily apparent. Despite the overwhelming needs and limited resources, the nursing presence as care was provided could indeed be called heroic.

The preparation of the professional nurses of South Africa in community health nursing and the leadership which they provide to the public is impressive. The high esteem in which the nurses are held by the public and the daily sacrifices that they make in time spent and the use of their own finances, as well as the solicitation of funds from others to meet care needs, re-enforced their altruism, a value highly regarded by nurses. The universality of nursing's ethos and the nurse's response to people in need of nursing services served as a common and reassuring bond.

Five of my colleagues from the Department of Nursing Science at the University of South Africa have provided case studies. In a country peopled by a large underserved black population, who for the most part are rural dwellers, a cultural mosaic presents itself for understanding and response as the healthcare needs of a nation in transition are met. The perspective that these colleagues provided lent an additional dimension that proved useful in our quest for increased understanding of the multifaceted dimensions of multiculturalism.

A lifetime of learning lies ahead. These case studies are presented to assist faculty and students in the continuing quest for offering nursing services that are sought out and preferred by the public.

Vernice D. Ferguson, RN, MA, FAAN, FRCN

ACKNOWLEDGMENTS

I am grateful to my colleagues who contributed to this book and to their deans in the Delaware Valley area schools of nursing, who recommended them to participate in the Independence Foundation funded project, "Preparing Nurses for America's Multicultural Future." Dean Norma Lang of the School of Nursing at the University of Pennsylvania has provided a supportive environment for my work as Senior Fellow occupying the Fagin Family Chair in Cultural Diversity throughout the course of this project.

Credit is due to Sylvia Johnson and Bonita Green, administrative assistants in the School of Nursing at the University of Pennsylvania, for their invaluable assistance in the preparation of this book. Thanks are also due to Eve Ferguson, my niece, who worked tirelessly with me in bringing this manuscript to completion.

V. D. F.

ABOUT THE AUTHOR

Vernice D. Ferguson, RN, MA, FAAN, FRCN, has had a long and distinguished career in federal service. Until her retirement in December 1992, she served as the Assistant Chief Medical Director for Nursing Programs of the Department of Veterans Affairs, the leadership role for more than 60,000 nursing personnel. Prior to this assignment, Ms. Ferguson was the Chief of the Nursing Department at the Clinical Center, the National Institutes of Health and served as Chief Nurse at the VA Medical Center, Madison, Wisconsin, and West Side Chicago, Illinois.

Ms. Ferguson is a fellow of the American Academy of Nursing and past president. She is an honorary fellow of the Royal College of Nursing of the United Kingdom, the second American nurse so honored. She is past president of Sigma Theta Tau International and is immediate past president of the International Society of Nurses in Cancer Care.

Her honors and awards are numerous, including the Lavinia Dock Prize for highest scholastic standing and honors in clinical practice from Bellevue–New York University, the Mary Mahoney Award of the American Nurses' Association, the Jean McVicar Outstanding Nurse Executive Award of the National League for Nursing, the Distinguished Service Award of the Department of Health and Human Services, and the Exceptional Service Award of the Department of Veterans Affairs. She is the recipient of two fellowships and seven honorary doctorates.

She is Senior Fellow in the School of Nursing at the University of Pennsylvania where she holds the Fagin Family Chair in Cultural Diversity.

CONTRIBUTORS

Marthie Bezuidenhout, D, Litt et Phil, in Nursing Management RN, is a Senior Lecturer, Department of Nursing Science at the University of South Africa. Areas of interest are human resources management, with special emphasis on labor relations health services. Dr. Bezuidenhout has conducted several short courses and workshops for service personnel in order to enhance their skills in managing labor relations.

Jane Brennan, DNSc, RN, is an Assistant Professor of Nursing in the College of Nursing at Widener University where she works primarily with undergraduate baccalaureate nursing students of diverse cultural and ethnic backgrounds. She is an ANA certified gerontological nurse with clinical interest in adult healthcare. Dr. Brennan serves as a volunteer with the Main Line Interfaith Hospitality Network for the homeless.

Elizabeth Dickason, EdD, RN, is an Assistant Professor of Nursing in the College of Nursing at Widener University. Her current research is focused on the health beliefs of employed women. While in the process of conducting a study of the breast cancer screening behaviors of women, Dr. Dickason is presenting programs to a diverse racial and ethnic group of women geared to facilitating their participation in breast self-exam, clinical breast exam, and mammography screening.

Shirlee Drayton-Hargrove, PhD, RN, is an Assistant Professor of Nursing in the Department of Nursing, College of Allied Health Professions at Temple University. She provides instruction on the graduate and undergraduate level. Dr. Drayton-Hargrove teaches the core graduate course, "Health Issues of Underserved and Diverse Populations" at the University. Her areas of expertise include multicultural issues, leadership, interaction analysis and rehabilitative aspects of care.

Sarie Human, M Cur, RN, is registered with the South African Nursing Council as General Nurse, Midwife, Psychiatric Nurse, Nurse Educator, and Nurse Manager. She serves as a lecturer in Community Nursing Science, Department of Nursing Science at the University of South Africa. Ms. Human is actively involved in various community health and community development programs.

Janet B. Foust, PhD, RN, is an Assistant Professor in the Nursing Department, College of Allied Health Professions at Temple University. She has served as consultant to the faculty consortium of Delaware Valley area schools of nursing on the Independence Foundation Grant focused on developing community focused and culturally sensitive case studies. Nurses' care planning across settings is an area of inquiry and publication for Dr. Foust.

Patricia Gerrity, PhD, RN, FAAN, is Associate Dean for Community programs in the School of Nursing at Allegheny University. She was the first Director of the LaSalle University Neighborhood Nursing Center, an innovative community nursing center initially funded by the Independence Foundation. Dr. Gerrity's graduate preparation in community health, health planning and city planning has served as a stimulus for significant grants that have supported her seminal contributions to grass roots, community-focused health and social welfare programs, and interdisciplinary leadership in teaching health administration, medical, and nursing students.

Katherine K. Kinsey, PhD, RN, FAAN, is an Associate Professor of Nursing at LaSalle University School of Nursing and Director of LaSalle University Neighborhood Nursing Center. She has been appointed to the Independence Foundation Endowed Chair in Nursing Education. Dr. Kinsey's eclectic research interests include program evaluation of Perinatal Home Visiting and Outreach Programs, HIV/AIDS related experiences of childbearing aged women and workplace violence. Other interests include building positive community collaboratives that facilitate Public Health Nursing students' learning in challenging culturally diverse urban settings. Dr. Kinsey has a broad and diverse clinical and educational background in public health nursing, such as hospice, home care, school health, policy development, and advocacy.

Helga Kirstein, MA (Cur), RN, is registered with the South African Nursing Council as General Nurse, Midwife, Psychiatric Nurse, Nurse Educator, and Community Health Nurse. She is a Lecturer, Department of Nursing Science at the University of South Africa. Mrs. Kirstein has been involved in South Africa's unique Health Care Train Project functioning in remote rural areas and providing primary healthcare, ophthalmic, dental, and other services to lower socioeconomic groups.

Maryanne McDonald, MSN, RN, is an Instructor in the Department of Nursing at Thomas Jefferson University. Ms. McDonald has extensive experience in community health nursing both in the field and in administration for more than 16 years. She has served on the board of directors of a number of community-oriented service organizations.

Frieda Outlaw, DNSc, RN, is an Assistant Professor and Program Director for Adult Psychiatric Mental Health and Special Populations at the University of Pennsylvania School of Nursing. Her post-doctoral training focused on the psychosocial adjustment to illness of African Americans with special emphasis on the role of religion and prayer as coping strategies. As a family therapist, Dr. Outlaw works with low-income families.

Dolores Patrinos, MA, RN, is an Assistant Professor in the Nursing Department, College of Allied Health Professions at Temple University. She was the principal investigator of a five-year project, "Nursing Career Opportunities Program" (NCOP) for students from under-represented minorities and economically disadvantaged backgrounds. Ms. Patrinos, while working with Open, Inc., in Philadelphia, taught community youths who were providing community health services to senior citizens in north Philadelphia.

Donna Faust Patterson, PhD, RN, is an Assistant Professor in the College of Nursing at Villanova University, Villanova, PA. Her clinical specialty is pediatric nursing. She has been a clinical instructor at the Children's Hospital of Philadelphia for 16 years. Her area of research is adolescent self-care behavior, specifically, self-care behaviors, cultural influences, and communication patterns surrounding menstruation. She has volunteered for school and church projects related to increasing cultural understanding.

JoAnne Reifsnyder, MSN, RN, OCN, is an Instructor in the Department of Nursing at Thomas Jefferson University in Philadelphia, Pennsylvania, a position that she has held for five years. Ms. Reifsnyder teaches courses in community health, ethics, and pain management. Ms. Reifsnyder oversees the operation of a walk-in health office at a large senior center in Philadelphia, where she has precepted nursing, occupational therapy, health education, and medical students. Ms. Reifsnyder is completing doctoral study at the School of Nursing at the University of Maryland.

Trinette Derkina Swanepoel, MA, RN, is registered with the South African Nursing Council as Midwife, Nurse Administrator, Nurse Educator, and Community Health Nurse. She is a Lecturer in the Department of Nursing Science, the University of South Africa, where she teaches community health nursing science. Her area of special interest is in informal support systems in home healthcare.

June Stewart, EdD, RN, CNA, is an Associate Professor in the Department of Nursing at Gwynedd Mercy College. She developed a course for advanced practice nursing with emphasis on the critical nature of cultural competence for nurse practitioners and clinical nurse specialists. Dr. Stewart has conducted workshops on cultural diversity in the healthcare delivery system and has taught classes on the impact of culture and race on clients' health-seeking behavior.

Donna Tartasky, PhD, RN, is Associate Dean for Special Projects and Partnerships in the School of Nursing at Southern Illinois University at Edwardsville, Edwardsville, Illinois. When the case studies were developed, she was an Assistant Professor in the College of Nursing at Villanova University where she taught community nursing at the undergraduate and graduate level. She served as a manuscript reviewer for *Public Health Nursing.* Dr. Tartasky is the recipient of two grants for a "Community Based Assessment of Adult Minority Asthmatics."

Dirk van der Wal, MA (Cur), RN, is registered with the South African Nursing Council as General Nurse, Community Health Nurse, Nurse Administrator, and Nurse Educator. He is a Lecturer in Nursing Education, Department of Nursing Science at the University of South Africa. Mr. van der Wal's area of inquiry is theory development in caring. Recently, he completed a study tour in the United States devoting his time to nursing's contributions to developments in this field.

Antonia M. Villarruel, PhD, RN, is an Assistant Professor at the University of Pennsylvania School of Nursing. Dr. Villarruel has had extensive research and practice experience with African American and Hispanic children and families. Her research includes studies in the area of pain assessment and management and promoting safe sexual behavior among adolescents. Dr. Villarruel serves as a research consultant to the National Coalition of Hispanic Health and Human Services Organizations and is president of the National Association of Hispanic Nurses.

PART ONE

INTRODUCTION

Chapter 1

CASE STUDIES

A Compelling New Direction

Vernice D. Ferguson

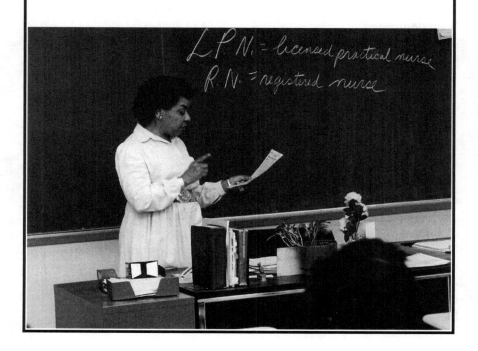

Through the Independence Foundation Grant, a faculty consortium, composed of faculty members in baccalaureate and higher degree programs in the greater Delaware Valley area schools of nursing, came together to discuss the increasing need to educate students for a different kind of nursing practice. In agreeing to develop case studies, we acknowledged that this approach should prove useful as we prepare nursing students to respond to the new realities in healthcare. A useful document that guided our deliberations as the case studies developed was *Essentials of College and University Education for Professional Nursing*, by the American Association of Colleges of Nursing.

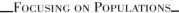

FOCUSING ON POPULATIONS

Meeting the healthcare needs of populations across the world is a daunting task. There is increasing recognition that resources are finite, even nonexistent for some needs. Along with the competing demands for use of available resources are the recognized needs and expectations of the population served.

In the United States, national goals have been proposed by the Department of Health and Human Services in its document, *Healthy People 2000: Health Promotion and Disease Prevention*. Five broad goals have been delineated:

1. Increase life expectancy to at least 78 years.
2. Increase the number of healthy years of life to at least 65.
3. Reduce infant mortality to no more than 7 per 1000 live births.
4. Decrease the disparity in life expectancy between white and minority populations to no more than 4 years.
5. Reduce disability caused by chronic conditions to no more than 7 percent of all people.

On the international level, the World Health Organization (WHO) proclaimed, "health for all by the year 2000." Although this is far from being realized, important progress is being made. The World Bank, the largest source of aid loans to developing countries, predicts that the average African baby born today can expect to live to age 54, while one born in 2030 should survive to age 63. The report states that action taken now on contraception and education can have a major influence after 2050. The study has also found that sending more girls to school and keeping them there results in fewer babies later. Education is clearly a priority for all people.

World meetings in the 1990s have focused on the well-being of children, women, economic development, environmental, and population issues. It is heartening to note that as major health and social welfare problems are confronted and as healthcare providers from the developed and developing world talk to each other, the traditional aid model of donor recipient dependency is giving way to education and participation.

The same strategy becomes the focus of nurses linking with people in the community to improve health and social welfare outcomes. *Empowerment* comes through *education* and *participation*. When the individual with the problem(s) participates in the resolution of the problems, a more lasting effect is achieved. Ownership is claimed and a more informed person emerges who is able to become a full partner as health outcomes improve.

A Climate of Change

Formidable challenges confront us as we prepare to accommodate the new realities in today's healthcare marketplace. Integrated healthcare systems emerge and managed care plans continue to expand, emphasizing lower healthcare costs by reducing the time for patient stays in hospitals. More healthcare, including nursing services, sophisticated therapies, and meal service, for example, take place in the home, neighborhood clinic, and hospital-based and group practice ambulatory care sites.

Most nurses who practice today were prepared to provide care primarily in hospitals. Consumers of healthcare services entered "our house" and, for the most part, received and accepted that which we provided within our walls and from our cultural perspective. The medical model, with the active provider and passive recipient, dominated. There were some variations evident as the behavioral (helping) model emerged in the delivery of rehabilitation and mental health services, including drug and alcohol programs.

Triggered by the goal of cost reduction in the delivery of healthcare services, we are continuing to witness a departure from acute, episodic hospital-based care to a continuum of care (Anderson, 1992). The community is coming into its own as services proliferate. With the shift in the funding priorities of leading healthcare focused foundations from acute to primary care, and with continued focus on the new healthcare professional who assures available, affordable, effective, and acceptable care, individuals and populations are being served in new ways and in new places. Attention to families and neighborhoods, community-based services, care of the elderly,

Table 1–1
GROWTH OF MINORITY POPULATIONS

Population	Make-Up of Total Population (Percent)	
	1990	2050
White	75	52
African American	12	23
Hispanic	9	14
Asian	3	10
Native American	1	1

Source: U.S. Census Bureau, 1992.

independent living for the physically and mentally disabled, substance abuse programs, and fostering changes toward healthier lifestyles have emerged as funding priorities (Sabatino, 1991).

Against these dramatic and continuing changes in the delivery of healthcare and its financing, we have come to realize that the population being served has changed as well. Along with the graying of America is the browning of America, signaling the rise of multiculturalism, and with it an increase in poverty levels, reflected all too often in lack of money, education, and good health.

At the turn of the 20th century in this nation of immigrants, the majority of new immigrants were of European ancestry. Now nearly one in four Americans is of African, Asian, Hispanic, or Native American ancestry. Among the major changes projected by the U.S. Census Bureau is the dramatic growth in the minority population (Table 1–1).

Table 1–2
MINORITIES IN SELECTED HEALTH PROFESSIONS

Occupation	Minorities (Percent of Total)	
	African American	Hispanic
Dentists	1.5	2.7
Pharmacists	3.4	3.2
Physicians	3.2	4.4
Psychologists	7.8	3.8
Registered Nurses	7.1	2.4

Source: U.S. Census Bureau, 1992.

Table 1–3
MINORITY REGISTERED NURSES

Estimates	
Black (non-Hispanic)	90,600
Hispanic	30,400
Asian/Pacific Islanders	76,000
American Indian/Alaskan Natives	10,000
Total	207,000 (9% of the 2.24 million registered nurses)

Source: DHHS—National Sample Survey, March 1992.

The growth in the number of minorities who choose healthcare careers has not kept pace with the general population. As a result, the diverse cultures do not have healthcare providers who adequately understand the client population (Table 1–2).

The number of minority registered nurses out of a population of more than two million nurses is appallingly low (Table 1–3). As a result, training the entire population of nurses to deal with an increasingly multicultural population is of paramount importance. Assuring increased sensitivity and greater cultural competence is a major criteria for healthcare educators.

CURRICULUM REFORM

Medical educators have begun to recognize that we need new knowledge that is more responsive to the new day. As we prepare healthcare professionals for a relevant practice now and into the 21st century, we are moving toward a new partnership between providers and recipients of care. Healthcare providers now become guests in the communities where individuals reside. This new relationship requires additional skills and knowledge.

A recent issue of the *Journal of the American Medical Association* (JAMA, September 4, 1996) focused on the need for change in medical education consonant with the rapid expansion of managed care. A century ago medical education recreated itself as a scientifically based discipline, yet it was never adequately extended to respond to the need to teach disease prevention as well as health promotion, requirements in managed care medicine. With increased emphasis on managing acute illness, the education of physicians never dealt adequately with the consequences of success in attending to acute illness. These successes have resulted in an expanding population of aging persons, the increasing prevalence and burden of chronic illness, as well as explosive growth in healthcare costs due to third-party payers who provided incentives for treatment over prevention and a healthcare delivery system that evolved around the hospital and episodic, technologically sophisticated care with very active providers and generally passive recipients of care.

Medical school training efforts are not responsive to the requirements of managed care. Despite profound changes in the healthcare delivery system and in education, medical students and resident physicians encounter a climate that is chilly toward primary care, evident from the perception that primary care tasks do not require high levels of expertise. Generalists may not be the best physicians to manage patients with serious illness. The quality of primary care research appears to be inferior to that in other fields.

Medical educators now recognize that as integrated health systems proliferate, physicians will be responsible for the health of a population and not just for individual patients. This requires knowledge in a number of areas including disease prevention and health promotion, epidemiology, social pathology and its consequences, community organization, and team building. Understanding the community in which people requiring services live is essential to successful interventions.

The parallels between changes required in medical education and nursing education are evident. Nurses have been prepared generally for practice in hospitals where the acute care model dominates. The majority of nurses are still working in hospitals. Presently, hospitals have changed their priorities from acute inpatient care to a continuum of care, from treating illness to maintaining wellness, and from filling beds to providing care at the appropriate level. Caring for individual patients has shifted to accountability for the health status of defined populations, hence new management skills are required of both physicians and nurses.

Historically, healthcare professional schools, nursing included, have not systematically incorporated cultural sensitivity into the educational programs or the healthcare delivery system. Not only does a change in the focus of the healthcare delivery system compel us to accelerate our learning in this arena, but the striking change in the demography of the population forces us to change as well. Now we must act and speak in a language with meanings that are relevant and acceptable to our new partners.

CASE STUDIES CONSIDERED

In schools of law and business, the case study is an integral part of the instructional process. In law schools, for instance, case law is presented beginning in the first year and continues through the three years, moving from simple to complex application. The student is challenged continually to think critically. Rather than focusing on remembering facts as case studies are presented, the student is expected to identify the problem (issue), elicit the facts, apply the facts to the law, and reach a conclusion.

There is value in using the case study approach in preparing nurses for work in the community where cultural factors take on increased meaning. Each case requires analysis and discussion. With all of the newness that surrounds us, an argument can be made for teaching strategies that are more responsive to today's reality.

New practice sites in the community and changing demographic patterns within them require the acquisition of new skills, new knowledge, and new attitudes. As new partnerships are formed and people are empowered to take greater responsibility for themselves, new teaching strategies must emerge in response to a markedly changed healthcare delivery system.

When the teacher engages the students in a case study approach, important learning takes place that is community-focused and culturally sensitive. As discussion unfolds during a case presentation, participants learn to enhance their communication skills, primarily actively listening to what others in the group are saying. This changes the focus, so essential in community-based care, to appreciating the perspective of others rather than defending the position that the proponent, whether teacher or learner, has put forth. New learning occurs for all participants through involvement in the discussion, sharing personal experiences, and reading background materials that add important dimensions. Just as in law school, students must be willing to accept criticism of any position assumed. Debate and open discussion enhance the ability to grow, to change, and to evaluate previously taken stances.

Case studies provide an unparalleled opportunity to explore a wide range of options. There is no absolute answer or right or wrong solution to a case presentation. As nurses become more present in the community and note the number and variety of problems presented by diverse individuals and populations, the "case" for using the case study approach is made. Its relevance is reflected in the number of useful solutions that are generated in response to each problem presented. Engaging the consumer as well as the provider in generating responses and valuing all of them increases the probability of more lasting problem resolution.

Both students and faculty have much to gain as the effect on culture and community are better understood when people are served. Case studies provide an opportunity for gaining new knowledge. Through them, the uniqueness of people and circumstances are recognized. Rather than making generalizations about a given situation, the case at hand is examined. The door is opened for a vast array of ideas. As problems emerge and a large number of cases are presented, new and more responsive remedies can be effected.

Case studies provide a useful way of responding to unique situations. This is especially useful in the multicultural arena where newness abounds. Learners should be challenged to confront their own beliefs, values, and biases, a necessary first step before acknowledging, accepting, adapting, and interacting with cultures and people in communities unlike their own.

The case study is an effective teacher/learner strategy that stimulates ideas through complex analysis of actual or hypothetical situations. Opportunities to apply theoretical principles abound.

Questions that should be considered when framing and resolving a case include:

1. What is happening? Why?
2. What are the problems? Why are these problems?
3. Where do they occur?
4. When do they occur?
5. How are they experienced?
6. Which problem(s) require attention? Why?
7. Which problems are of minimal consequence?
8. Which problems can be ignored? Why?
9. Who is affected by the problem(s)?
10. What are the basic underlying issues?
11. What are the areas of agreement? Conflict?
12. What can be done to resolve the problem(s)?
13. Are the resolutions acceptable for the problems presented?
14. Are the resolutions realistic—culturally, economically, politically?
15. What is the "best" solution? Why?
16. How will the action course be evaluated?

The Value of Case Studies

In a clinical practice discipline such as nursing, case studies offer limitless opportunities for exploring viable options to enrich the practice. People with all of their complexity are at the center of nursing's purpose. The variations and richness of responses that are possible when case studies are used provide students with a valuable approach to enhance critical thinking and creativity.

In the preparation of professional nurses for practice, the American Association of Colleges of Nursing has delineated twelve abilities that should be acquired (see pp. 4–5). Included is the ability to evaluate information and think critically and creatively, a skill essential to the deliberative process when case studies are used. Knowledge is required coupled with an attitude of inquiry, thereby assuring greater skill in application of nursing and healthcare services.

What are the characteristics of critical thinking that become useful in the development and use of case studies for the baccalaureate nursing student and the faculty member guiding their use? A restatement of the work of Loucine Huckabay, PhD, RN (1990), University of Illinois College of Nursing, and discussion at the Eighth Annual and Sixth International Conference on Critical Thinking and Educational Reform (1986), Sonoma State University, California, as well as reflections from the author, lend themselves to the enhancement of critical thinking through the use of case studies in a multicultural context.

1. Think actively.
2. Carefully explore a situation or an issue.
3. Be open to new ideas and different viewpoints.
4. Be aware of your own biases, perceptions, and assumptions.
5. Discuss ideas in an organized way.
6. Support your views with reason and evidence.
7. Think in terms of concepts.
8. Employ relevant principles in problem solving.
9. Offer appropriate arguments to support conclusions.
10. Withhold judgments without evidence.
11. Separate the reality that is presented from your own viewpoint.
12. Evaluate the credibility of sources used to justify a point of view.
13. Clarify and critique what is presented for evidence.
14. Distinguish relevant from irrelevant observations and significant from trivial observations and facts.
15. Transfer ideas to new contexts and situations.
16. Make plausible inferences and distinguish conclusions from the reasoning that supports them.
17. Search for alternatives or options.
18. Recognize and deal with contradictions.
19. Test and refine generalizations.

Giving voice to the student using creative problem-solving techniques is not unlike giving voice to the consumers of nursing services. In each instance, helpful and acceptable solutions to problems are sought as people are empowered to take control of their lives.

Creativity is also required to optimize critical thinking. Albrecht defines creativity "as the process of producing new, novel, and occasionally useful ideas." Some of the methods associated with creative thinking are useful as students and faculty use case studies. Among these methods are brainstorming and synectics. Workable solutions for individuals and families are achieved as healthcare problems are identified and resolved in ways that are acceptable to the consumers of nursing services.

Brainstorming was one of the first creative thinking methods developed. Through group problem-solving techniques, all ideas are considered without judging any of them. This becomes a useful technique when working in the multicultural arena. Using this technique, a wide range of ideas is generated, increasing the likelihood that workable solutions to problems will be realized. Stimulating the imagination to propose alternative solutions in an uninhibited environment not only engages student and faculty in dialogue, but fosters an environment that is conducive to mutually respectful conduct between the recipient of nursing service and the provider.

Synectics is defined as the study of creative processes especially as applied to the solution of problems by a group of diverse individuals. When people of varied backgrounds meet to problem solve, they bring with them a richness. In an environment that is unrestricted, the exercise of imagination and the correlation of disparate elements is encouraged.

A Case Study in Progress

During my interaction with university nursing students, one of them offered a real-life situation that was troublesome. She felt inadequate to resolve the situation to her satisfaction. This case provides a potent example of what one confronts in providing responsive services in an increasingly multicultural society. No attempt is made to solve the dilemma. This case study lends itself to creative problem-solving techniques. Each time that the same case is presented to students, it is gratifying to note their observations of subtle and overt nuances that surface as well as the dynamic solutions offered for the problems identified.

Case Study
Cultural Sensitivity

S is a sophomore from Pakistan. She does have some family in the United States, but her immediate family is still in Pakistan. S. is a tiny "frail" looking person who is very homesick. As a result of her homesickness and need for attention, she has had many "health" problems. Some of them appear to be more psychological than physical.

This semester S. has had a chest cold that she just can't shake and while she doesn't need to see the doctor two or three times a week as in the past, she is audibly congested and feels sick. After several weeks of treatment with no results, S.'s uncle, who lives in the United States, came to the health clinic to discuss the problem with the staff. The doctor refused to deal with the uncle, stating that this was an issue between himself (the doctor) and the patient S. The uncle was unmoved and pushed further stating that the two of them could discuss the situation "man to man." The doctor eventually did speak to the uncle briefly, but later told the staff that S.'s problems stem from being dominated by male influences in her life and that he (the doctor) could cure one-half of her ills if he could teach her to have some backbone.

The saga continues with S. getting a package from home, filled with herbal remedies that her mother thought might help her get over her cold. S., thinking she was being responsible, brought them with her on her next visit to see the doctor and asked how she could use these in conjunction with the medicine he was giving her. The doctor dismissed the herbal remedies with the statement, "You can use them if you want, but they will not do anything for you." He then later joked with the health clinic staff that he knew the package from home was bound to arrive, because "all of those South Asian cultures like to throw in a folk remedy or two." S. continues to come to the health clinic regularly for a combination of ailments and homesickness.

- If you were the doctor in the health clinic and S. presented herself to you, how would you have managed her care? Justify your actions.
- If you were a health clinic staff member (a nurse), what would you have done?

Case Study
In and Beyond the Emergency Room

A community health practicum can enrich the student's understanding and responsiveness to individuals who are being served in a variety of ambulatory case settings including the emergency room. The impact of lifestyle and the environment must be considered as care is provided. These considerations are often dramatic in the emergency room setting yet may be daunting for the student. Understanding the cultural dimension becomes crucial in the provision of responsive care. The patient's appearance in the emergency room is often the beginning of a long pathway to the best health possible, as social and clinical pathways converge.

The case of J.M. reminds us of the ever-expanding opportunities to demonstrate nursing's effectiveness through astute assessments and purposeful interactions with many partners in care. J.M., who is 7-years-old, is brought to the medical emergency room by her grandmother after she began a crying spell at home and appeared to be in respiratory distress. After being examined and medically cleared, the family was referred to the Psychiatric Emergency Services.

J.M. is a small, thin African American child who is dressed in ill-fitting clothes, and her braids look uncombed. She is quick to engage in a conversation with the nurse and seems to be older than her chronological age. She talks about her mother whom she rarely sees, and about her grandmother who is "good to her" but drinks. Her affect is sad as she describes her community and living next door to a "crack house." She describes her house as without water. "I bring water up from the basement and use it for cooking and washing." Her grades are good at school and she seldom misses a day. She describes her relationship with other children as strained. "They laugh at my clothes and my hair, and leave me out of games." When asked if she is suicidal, she states, "I can't do that until I am old enough to think about an effective way."

1. What are the developmental tasks of a 7-year-old child?
2. What are some of the sociocultural influences that need to be assessed?
3. How would you interview to obtain information about her self-identity?
4. How would you assess the functioning of her support system?
5. Identify risk factors in the family system.
6. Identify strengths.
7. What is some of the social-cultural "noise" that might get in the way as the nurse attempts to implement the nursing process?

_____REFERENCES_____

Albrecht, K. (1987). *The creative corporation*. Homewood, IL: Dow Jones-Irwin.

American Association of Colleges of Nursing (AACN). (1986). *Essentials of college and university education for professional nursing* (final report). Washington, DC: Author.

Anderson, H. (1992). Hospitals seek new ways to integrate health care. *Hospitals, 66*(7), 26–36.

Beyond the melting pot. (1990, April 9). *Time*, 28–31.

Davis, G. A., & Scott, J. A. (1971). *Training creative thinking*. New York: Holt.

Division of Nursing, Bureau of Health Professions, Health Resources and Services Administration DHHS. (February 1994). *The registered nurse population 1992*. Washington, DC: U.S. Government Printing Office.

Entire issue. (1996, September 4). *JAMA. 276*(9).

Farson, R. (1969, September 6). How could anything that feels so bad be good? *Saturday Review of Literature*, 20–21.

Ferguson, V. (1994). The future of nursing. In O. Strickland & D. Fishman (Eds.), *Nursing issues in the 1990s*. Albany, NY: Delmar.

Garver, E. (1986). Critical thinking: Them and us. A response to Arnold Aaron's critical thinking and baccalaureate curriculum. *Liberal Education, 72*, 245–252.

Giger, J., & Davidhizar, R. (1991). *Transcultural nursing: Assessment and intervention*. St. Louis: Mosby Year Book.

Koop, C. E. (1996). Manage with care. *Time, 148*(14), 69.

Leininiger, M. (1981). Transcultural nursing: Its progress and its future. *Nursing and Health Care, 11*(7), 365–370.

Levenstein, A. (1976). Effective change requires change agent. *Hospitals, 50*, 71–74.

Lipson, J., Dibble, S., & Minarik, P. (Eds.). (1996). *Culture and nursing care: A pocket guide*. San Francisco: University of California San Francisco Nursing Press.

Lipson, J. G., & Meleis, A. I. (1985). Culturally appropriate care: The case of immigrants. *Topics in Clinical Nursing, 7*(3), 48–56.

Maryland's Integrated Health Service Expands. (1996, October 22). *The Washington Post*, C2.

Miller, M. A., & Malcolm, N. S. (1990). Critical thinking in the nursing curriculum. *Nursing and Health Care, 11*(2), 67–73.

Sabatino, F. (1991). Foundations' funding priorities shift from acute to primary care. *Hospitals, 65*(11), 34, 36–37.

Stice, J. E. (Ed.). (1987). *Developing critical thinking and problem-solving abilities.* San Francisco: Jossey-Bass.

Tappen, R. M. (1983). *Nursing and leadership: Concepts and practices.* Philadelphia: Davis.

Thomas, E. (Ed.). (1995). *Race and ethnicity in America: Meeting the challenge in the 21st century.* Washington, DC: Taylor and Francis.

Chapter 2

A Consultant's Perspective

Janet B. Foust, PhD, RN

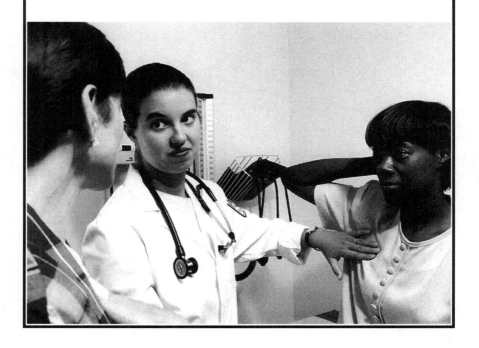

COMMENTARY

Vernice D. Ferguson

Dr. Foust served as consultant to the Independence Foundation Project, "Preparing Nurses for America's Multicultural Future." She makes a strong case for the role of nurses as advocates. We are reminded that advocacy is crucial to the well-being of vulnerable people.

Nursing care has become an essential part of community-based health services. Hence, nurse educators must assure that students in baccalaureate nursing programs acquire the necessary skills to provide culturally acceptable care. Communication skills, which include active listening, risk assessment, potential problem identification, and early intervention are to be mastered by nurses as individuals. Families and communities participate fully in health promotion and disease prevention endeavors. Fostering client independence, health education and health promotion are often overlooked or minimized in the acute care setting. The students' community health experience offers an unparalleled opportunity to students to become comfortable in the provision of community-oriented, culturally competent care—a requirement now and into the 21st century.

Healthcare is changing at a dynamic and almost explosive rate. Basic assumptions have been redefined and different priorities have been established. The most obvious change has been the emphasis on cost effectiveness of care. There is a stronger focus on community-based care. Professional nurses remain central to any healthcare delivery system, and as such, are in pivotal roles to positively influence patient care in a variety of settings. Nurse educators must address emerging issues through curriculum re-design, selection of clinical experiences, and identified student outcomes. The American Association of Colleges of Nursing (AACN) (1986) recommends cultivating twelve specific competencies, including:

1. Communication skills that demonstrate knowledge and critical thinking;
2. Analytical thinking;
3. Comprehension of a second language to enhance culturally competent care;
4. Understanding of other cultural traditions and associated values;
5. Use of mathematical skills and information technologies;
6. Use of behavioral and biological sciences to aid in understanding the nature and functions of communities;
7. Comprehending the physical world;
8. Perceiving historical and current perspectives;
9. Learning about social, political, and economic views necessary to resolve societal problems;
10. Understanding human spirituality and its interrelatedness to health, culture, behavior, and healing;
11. Recognizing the positive influence of the fine arts on creative expression; and
12. Understanding human values as a basis of personal philosophy and professional life (AACN, 1986).

The AACN report underscores the importance of baccalaureate education as the essential foundation needed to provide professional nursing practice in the current healthcare environment.

One of the most profound influences on healthcare delivery has been the cost of services and the more recent and dramatic efforts to manage these expenses. The current emphasis on delivering cost-effective care has produced extensive changes in healthcare delivery. One outcome has been the increased need for community-based care. People are discharged from hospitals more quickly than in the past. Often they have continuing, complex healthcare needs that must be met by the individual, family, or community services. As a result, the demand for nursing care in the community is more acute than ever before. Community-based care demands that the nurse incorporate the clients' values, culture, and environment into any treatment plan. Participation by the people most directly affected by a treatment plan is central to effective patient care management and is most appropriate in community-based nursing care.

Consultant Role

Working as a consultant on an Independence Foundation Grant to develop culturally sensitive and community-based case studies, I listened, read, and learned about the experiences of providing culturally sensitive care in a variety of communities. It is not surprising that there are differences and unique aspects to each community. However, there are also similarities in delivering professional nursing care to diverse people/populations. Many of the consortium discussions focused on how nurse educators need to cultivate cultural competence during the students' community health experiences. It is an ideal time to integrate issues of caring for culturally diverse and underserved populations into the actions of nursing. One of the most striking themes from our discussions of culturally sensitive care in the community was the importance of communication skills as a means to reach out and establish trust with people of different cultural backgrounds and lifestyles. Culturally competent communication reflects an attitude of critical thinking that demonstrates an openness to learn from others, view situations from another person's perspective, and use acquired knowledge of cultural traditions and values. It requires someone to suspend one's own values and judgments in order to actively listen to another person's experience and situation. Culturally competent communication means that nurses must put aside any ethnocentrism so that they can make accurate and sensitive assessments based on the individual, family, or community—not predetermined assumptions. As individuals, families, and communities, people adopt selected values, rituals, and aspects of their own heritage that must be acknowledged. An accurate assessment is the first step to developing an effective and culturally appropriate plan of care.

The process of actively listening and establishing trust integrates the seven essential professional nursing values identified by the AACN (1986): altruism, equality, esthetics, freedom, human dignity, justice, and truth. These values have corresponding attitudes and behaviors. For example, human dignity is associated with attitudes of consideration, empathy, humaneness, kindness, respectfulness, trust, and behaviors safeguarding the client's right to privacy, addressing clients as they prefer, maintaining confidentiality, and treating others with respect regardless of background. Sensitivity and therapeutic communication with others are cognitive-based skills that demonstrate the values, knowledge, and competencies expected of professional nurses.

Another important consideration in community-based care is the role clients play in their own care. The hospital setting is a controlled setting with many well-established routines and a primary focus on the acute event leading to hospitalization. The urgency and acuity of the patient's healthcare problems take priority, often to the exclusion of other less-urgent but important healthcare issues. For example, there are times when someone is admitted to a hospital without a primary healthcare provider. In a setting that reacts to acute problems, finding a primary healthcare provider to improve post-hospital care is improbable. In contrast, community-based care occurs in a setting controlled more by the client where routines are adapted to the environment and the focus of care is on recuperation, recovery, and regaining independence and health. Unlike the acute care setting where nurses and physicians are present and available 24 hours a day, nurses in the community must rely on the clients to follow through with instructions and treatments. This creates a more collaborative relationship between the nurses and clients, focused on mutually set health goals.

The community is an ideal setting for students to see and respond to some of the objectives that address management of chronic illness, improving functional abilities, as well as health promotion and disease prevention. These issues are more clearly seen when caring for people in their own environments. Nurses providing care in the community are alert to the most urgent clinical issues; they facilitate client independence, health education, and health promotion that are necessarily overlooked in more acute situations. The nurses also have the opportunity to assess family interactions, understand the nature and availability of formal and informal resources, as well as the influence of the physical environment on the client's health.

An increasingly pivotal role of professional nursing care is to encourage and facilitate health promotion and disease prevention. Consequently, risk assessment is an implicit skill that uses scientific knowledge and astute assessment skills to determine appropriate health goals, interventions and/or avoid anticipated problems. Risk assessment, potential problem identification, and early intervention are essential to effective health promotion and disease prevention interventions. Health promotion and disease prevention are important areas for nursing to embrace in a cost-effective healthcare climate. It is an opportunity to demonstrate what professional nursing care does well—avoid problems through client education and improve coordination of care across settings. Furthermore, as the impetus grows for more population-based health planning, nurses' competency with risk identification, environmental assessments, as well as health promotion and disease prevention strategies, will become fundamental. Effective health promotion or disease prevention strategies require a cultural assessment of client values and resources.

Patient advocacy is another essential competency of professional nursing focused on the goal of justice and fair allocation of resources (AACN, 1986). Specifically, the rapidity of reorganization amid healthcare reform and diminishing resources underscores the importance of patient advocacy in professional nursing practice. From the clients' perspectives, one effect of the many simultaneous changes is that healthcare routines, resources, and access have been disrupted. An essential component of fair and appropriate healthcare delivery is access to providers, resources, and care. For those individuals who are vulnerable, these changes magnify their difficulties in obtaining needed care.

Advocacy incorporates the values of justice, scientific knowledge, critical thinking abilities, and communication skills to intervene on behalf of a client. The advocacy role of nurses has been demonstrated in the expert practice of clinical nurse specialists and nurse practitioners. There is no substitute for experience and acquired knowledge as a basis for being an effective advocate. However, nurse educators should not leave to chance the development of such an essential clinical competency.

Specifically, nurses at all levels need to cultivate the necessary communication skills to present and substantiate clinical judgments or decisions to others in a manner that is sound, persuasive, and offers guidance in patient care. For people who are vulnerable, advocacy is crucial to their well-being. Furthermore, in order to provide culturally competent and appropriate care, nurses must be able to make a case to other healthcare providers and agencies to obtain the needed care for clients when they cannot do so themselves. Other aspects of nursing advocacy are providing guidance through the health care system and translating events and recommendations to the clients. Some people are unfamiliar with the culture of American healthcare and need assistance to learn what steps should be taken and in what order. This problem is magnified for individuals who have recently emigrated and require help with the language. Other people requiring nurse advocates may be familiar with the healthcare system, but different values or alternative healthcare practices generate conflict or miscommunication. In all these instances, clients need nurses as advocates who can facilitate client access to quality care.

REFERENCES

American Association of Colleges of Nursing (AACN). (1986). *Essentials of college and university education for professional nursing* (final report). Washington, DC: Author.

U.S. Public Health Service. (1990). *Healthy people 2000: National health promotion and disease prevention objectives* (Doc. # PHS91-50213). Washington, DC: U.S. Government Printing Office.

PART TWO

CASE STUDIES

Chapter 3

Inner City Healthcare

Variations on a Theme

Frieda Outlaw

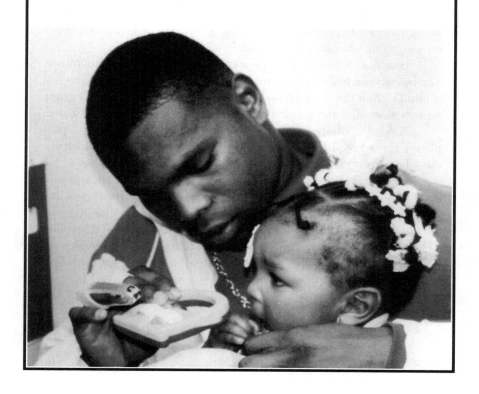

Vernice D. Ferguson

The two case studies presented by Dr. Outlaw demonstrate dramatically what can be achieved when a culturally competent nurse provides care for two clients and their family members. The strategies used to achieve significant and positive health outcomes are useful to consider when treating culturally diverse people.

In the first case study, *joining* becomes an important first step as care is provided, followed by the *assessment* phase and finally, *termination.* In the second case study, *cognitive restructuring* proved an effective technique as the nurse related to this African American client.

Both case studies display *the* fundamental requirement when providing service to people. It is respect—respect for person, home, and living circumstances. To provide the most responsive and acceptable community-based, culturally competent care, the nurse must work within the confines of the family and the client's belief system.

People being served have stories to tell. Telling these stories and being listened to provide valuable insights to be incorporated in the nurses' comprehensive plan of care.

How easy it is to stereotype members of a particular subculture. The two strikingly different families, their lifestyles and environments, remind us that the uniqueness of individuals and members of a group must be regarded and accommodated as care is planned and provided.

Making a difference in the community as culturally diverse people are served requires that the nurse grow constantly. New knowledge must be acquired, along with the requirement to examine that which was known and used in the past to determine whether or not it is still appropriate. Being knowledgeable about community resources and using them appropriately is critical to the successful interventions of the nurse. Nursing knowledge, as well as techniques gleaned from other fields, is imperative for effective nursing care. Dr. Outlaw provides superb examples of how it all comes together on behalf of those whom nursing serves.

An Inner-City, Multigenerational African American Family

—————————————OBJECTIVES—————————————

1. Discuss race, ethnicity, socioeconomic status, and cultural issues related to the treatment of many poor inner-city African American families.
2. Discuss issues related to working with multigenerational, poor, inner-city African American families.
3. Discuss strategies to engage all members of the family in the patient's plan of care when the nurse is of a different racial or ethnic cultural group and/or is of different socioeconomic conditions from the family.

*M*rs. M. is a 74-year-old African American woman who was referred to the psychiatric consultant of the Visiting Nurse Association after she refused to have the current medical nurse visit her anymore. Mrs. M. had been referred to the Visiting Nurse Association because she has chronic pulmonary disease, uncontrolled hypertension, insulin dependent diabetes, and a history of major depression. It had been noted by Mrs. M.'s primary physician that every time she becomes upset and stressed, usually about family matters, she has a medical crisis and is admitted to the hospital by way of the emergency room.

Mrs. M. moved to Philadelphia after separating from her husband over thirty years ago. However, she maintained a relationship with him until his death four years ago. She often talked of her "sorrow" about his death. Mrs. M. is the mother of five children: two boys and three girls. All of her children are living, although one of her sons is terminally ill with cancer. Mrs. M. frequently spoke of the sadness she feels about not being able to visit her ill son who lives in another city. She was concerned about her son because she has not been able to determine the nursing home where he was placed for care by his estranged wife. As a result, she has not been able to talk to him on the telephone for over two years. During the nursing visits, Mrs. M. often talked about going to visit her son although other family members, when out of her presence, would say that she would not be able to make the trip for several reasons, including lack of financial resources as well as not knowing where to find her son.

Mrs. M. lives in a small, three-bedroom row house with two of her daughters, one son, and a grandson. Mrs. M. and both daughters have their own separate rooms. On several occasions, her son was observed sleeping on a sofa bed in the dining room. It is unclear where the grandson, who is 22, sleeps. Mrs. M.'s son who lives in the house has a history of drug and alcohol abuse, and one of the daughters has a history of mental illness. Neither sibling has been able to find employment, which creates a stressful situation in the household.

The family members were all organized to participate in the management of their mother's diabetes and hypertension. Her son's girlfriend was also a vital part of the daily management of Mrs. M.'s healthcare. Mrs. M. took no direct responsibility for managing her own care.

The chaotic family dynamics were evident in the way responsibilities for Mrs. M.'s care were organized. For example, one of the daughters was responsible for managing her mother's medicine, including the insulin. Her son was responsible for managing the food preparation for his mother. The two siblings, however, were in frequent conflict and had difficulty talking with one another. Therefore, there was very little coordination between the two about the management of their mother's diabetes. Mrs. M.'s blood sugar was routinely very labile as a result of this lack of coordination and because of her noncompliance with her dietary regime. Often she was eating cookies and drinking sugared commercial ice tea or soda when the consultant arrived. In contrast, some visit days she would not have eaten anything but a slice of toast with her morning insulin. She and her son often engaged in heated arguments about her eating patterns. He frequently accused his mother of not cooperating with him about matters related to food. Sometimes they would not have enough insulin, and the visiting nurse would spend considerable time getting prescription renewals from the primary physician.

The girlfriend was responsible for monitoring Mrs. M.'s blood sugar level and blood pressure daily. She kept a record and was often present to discuss the results with the nurse. She had to be considered a part of the extended support system because Mrs. M. was very accepting of the girlfriend's input about her care. Therefore, in order to join with her, the visiting nurse consultant had to recognize and value this extended family constellation. Mrs. M.'s oldest daughter lived in another part of the city. Her role appeared to be that of peacemaker and ultimate family authority when the tension between the siblings who lived in the house became too great.

Often when the visiting nurse consultant would arrive at the home, Mrs. M. would be upstairs in her daughter's room in bed, head covered, with all the lights off. She would describe being sad and anxious. Her youngest daughter would be working; however, her son and other daughter would both be present for the visit although they did not talk to one another. The girlfriend would arrive shortly after the nurse to provide patient information.

QUESTIONS

1. As a visiting nurse who is racially, ethnically, culturally, and/or socioeconomically different from the patient, what is the most important initial therapeutic intervention to make with the patient and his/her family?
2. Describe at least two problems common to urban poor people of color that impact on the coping and compliance of this patient.
3. Discuss the role that extended kinship network relationships play in the management of a patient of color who has a chronic illness.
4. Discuss two characteristics of the family in this case study using the broad guidelines describing the cultural norms and values of many African American families.

ANALYSIS AND DISCUSSION

This case study describes the barriers and obstacles that many poor, urban, African American extended kinship family networks experience when the family has a member with a chronic disease. Mrs. M., the patient, has a long history of physical and mental problems. Most of her children either live with her or close by, and the extended-family dynamics have both positive and negative or dysfunctional qualities. A vital function of the psychiatric visiting nurse is to assess the positive and dysfunctional patterns of the extended family network and to determine how these patterns are impacting on the health of the patient.

Comprehensive planning by the nurse includes first recognizing the clinical implications of including extended family networks in the patient's treatment plan. It also requires that the nurse recognize that many times these families include in their networks persons who are not a member of the family genealogically, but who are otherwise related to a member of the family and function as members of the family. Their roles and position in the family must also be considered when plans for the care of the patient are being made.

Boyd-Franklin (1989) describes the centrality of reciprocity, the sharing of resources by extended African American family networks, as a crucial survival method used by families when resources may be limited. In this case study, the son's girlfriend provided a necessary supportive reciprocal function. Because she had been trained as a nurse aide, and because she worked at night, she was able to accompany Mrs. M. to all of her doctor's appointments and served as the liaison between the doctor and the other family members. She was also responsible for keeping detailed records of the patient's blood sugar level and blood pressure. Her ability to take on the task of recording vital patient data and escorting the patient to the doctor relieved other members of the family of these responsibilities. In turn, she was supported and respected in the family as a person critical to the care of Mrs. M. In fact, when the nurse initially visited the patient, she was introduced to S., the girlfriend, and her role was described to the nurse by the patient. Therefore, the care plan for Mrs. M. would include a role for S. as a way of modeling reciprocity by the nurse and as a way of joining the family system in a manner that demonstrates respect for their way of functioning.

Other strategies to be developed for working with this family include joining with them in a way that demonstrates respect for the family. Munichin (1974) and Boyd-Franklin (1989) believe that when working with families of color, such as African American families, the joining process can be the most difficult aspect. The M. family had previously dismissed several nurses because they felt that the nurses were disrespectful. They later described instances in which a new nurse would visit Mrs. M. and on the first visit begin to tell the family what they could and could not do in the house. For example, Mrs. M. had asthma and should not be exposed to cigarette smoke. However, several of the children who lived with her smoked cigarettes. One of the visiting nurses demanded that the family members refrain from smoking in the house because of their mother's asthma.

While the attempt to eliminate as much second-hand smoke from the patient's presence was the medically appropriate path to take, the timing of the educational intervention was inappropriate. It is imperative that the nurse establish a relationship with the patient and the extended family before giving directives to change their behavior. This type of joining can take several visits in which the nurse demonstrates respect for the family she or he is visiting. For example, many times nurses call patients by their first name. This subtle, but significant, informal behavior may be the nurse's attempt at being friendly; however, many elderly African American patients may experience such behavior as disrespectful since many of them associate it with the dehumanizing disrespect of adult African American women and men that they experienced in the past: that is, failure to address them appropriately as "Miss," "Mrs.," or "Mr." *because* they were African American.

Joining with extended African American families is the first step in providing care for the identified patient. Joining consists of conveying to each family member that their input is vital. For example, initially S., the girlfriend, was sometimes intrusive in the nurse's interactions with Mrs. M. Observing S.'s behavior, the nurse, instead of competing with her, included her in the care planning by recognizing her very useful contribution of keeping the patient's data. Second, it is vital that the nurse convey respect for the family, their home, and living circumstances. Many homes that nurses visit may be modest and in some cases unkempt. They also are often in neighborhoods that are drug infested and have many rundown or abandoned buildings. One strategy by which to engage the patient is to talk about what the neighborhood was like when the family first moved into it. Often, elderly family members will discuss what it was like to integrate a neighborhood and provide other interesting historical facts that give the nurse insight into family beliefs, values, and coping strategies.

According to Boyd-Franklin (1989), after the joining phase, comes the assessment phase in which most of the work involves observing family dynamics, so that ideas about what is going on in the family can be developed. It is an ongoing process and many times the hypotheses that are first formulated will change over time with more family observation and information gathering. For instance, Mrs. M.'s son was responsible for preparing her daily meals while his sister was responsible for managing her medicines. It was clear early on that the two siblings did not coordinate their assigned functions due to tensions in their relationship. As a result, Mrs. M.'s blood sugar was often very labile and unstable.

Observation of the family communicational pattern is important for the nurse to note so that, as she becomes more joined with the family members, she can develop strategies to intervene to change a dysfunctional family communication pattern. Many times strained family patterns of communication often shield long-standing family secrets or disputes. Families of color, African American families in particular, have been found to be quite suspicious of healthcare providers, thus family secrets are usually not disclosed until the family feels very connected to the nurse.

The visiting nurse is responsible for teaching the patient and the family members about the management of the patient's illness. Skilled nursing assessment requires the nurse to monitor the situation in order to determine when the time is right to engage the family in problem solving related to the patient's care. Additionally, the nurse must present herself/himself as nonjudgmental if she or he is to create an atmosphere in which all family members will feel comfortable enough to share their fears and concerns. When family secrets and problems are shared readily with the nurse by family members, effective interventions can be developed. Often if the nurse is of a different race, ethnic group, or socioeconomic status than the patient, it is at this time in the relationship that she or he can raise issues of race, ethnicity, or class. This approach to patient management acknowledges obvious differences between and among people. Encouraging a discussion of the obvious assists the nurse in establishing credibility with the patient and the family.

Another feature of this case involves working with the patient and her family to help recognize and intervene in her depression. This begins the problem-solving phase during which problems are identified and plans made to intervene therapeutically. As a result of her depression, the patient was very demanding and critical of her family. She refused to take any responsibility for the management of her care and often would be found lying in her bed with the lights off and the covers over her head when the nurse arrived. According to the family members, this pattern of behavior had been used by the patient throughout her life when she was stressed or depressed. Family members expressed frustration and anger about the demands she constantly made on them.

Many African American families have a collective focus because that is what they have needed to survive the pressures of invidious racial discrimination. In this case, the individual family members need to be coached on how to work with their mother in a more therapeutic manner. Setting limits and boundaries for elderly people in African American cultures can often bring conflict within individual family members and within the group because the cultural norm is that the elderly embody the wisdom of the group and are to be respected. Most experts who work with African American families believe that, in order to facilitate change in these families, the health-care provider must work within the belief systems of the family.

In the case of Mrs. M., one of the interventions used by the nurse during each visit was to remark on how well her children took care of her and to offer the assessment that she must have been a good mother in order to have received this much loyalty from them. In making this point on many occasions, the nurse was able to suggest to Mrs. M. that the caregivers were working very hard to care for her and could use a break. Once she was comfortable that her children were "doing right" by her, she agreed to go to a program for frail elderly like herself three days a week.

This day program allowed her adult caregiver children to focus on some of their needs. For example, her son started looking for a job. It was clear, however, that if he found a job the system would be in chaos again because Mrs. M. often remarked that she did not know what she would do if her son was not there to "take care of her." In this case, the long-term goal would be to work on the enmeshment issues that the family system demonstrated and to assist Mrs. M. in taking more responsibility for her own care. In addition, it was important to intervene in her loneliness and social isolation by engaging her in social networks beyond the home by using community resources such as a church and local senior citizen center. In urban communities such as the one in which Mrs. M. lives, it is imperative that healthcare providers have knowledge of available resources of this kind.

It is also important to form a relationship with the adult children in the home so that they become comfortable with you as the healthcare provider. This relationship requires that the provider enter the system in a nonjudgmental way while recognizing the contributions that all are making. Establishing trusting relationships with all the family members allows the nurse to suggest new approaches to the patient's care once trust has been established.

After Mrs. M. had been enrolled in a program for the frail elderly that she attended three times a week, the nurse was in the termination phase with the patient and her family when both the patient and the daughter started asking problematic questions such as, "Where can my mother get a telephone with large numbers so she can call for help fast if she needs to?" Instead of answering what, on the surface, seemed an informational question, the nurse explored the subtle meaning of what the daughter was asking. Probing, because trust had been established, the nurse discovered that the brother who lived in the house and was responsible for much of his mother's care had started to drink again and had been somewhat verbally abusive toward the mother over the weekend. Although both the mother and the daughter denied that the son had ever been physically abusive to the mother, they were nevertheless concerned.

As a first step, the nurse educated the two women about the resources available to them and reinforced the information with written materials. She also helped them to talk about their fears and concerns. While the best intervention for this family would have been to have a family session where the issues of verbal and physical abuse could have been discussed, the family was unwilling to do this. However, the nurse used the relationship she had developed with the son to talk to him about his stresses, concerns, and frustrations. He shared that he was particularly frustrated about not being able to get a job. After validating his frustration, he was encouraged to re-connect with Alcoholics Anonymous and was directed to contact the job bank at the Urban League.

Visiting nurses have to view the family as a whole. Therefore, they can-not provide services to only the patient and expect that the patient's health-care needs will be met. A multisystem approach, in which the nurse conceptualizes and plans interventions that target multiple levels and mul-tiple systems, has to be developed when providing care for African Amer-ican patients.

In this case study, multilevel approaches included developing a relation-ship with all family members who were involved in the life of the patient. A relationship with an extended family member who had a vital responsibility in the management of the patient's diabetes and hypertension was included in the multisystem approach. The patient, until recently, had been an active member of her church. That social system was included very prominently in the nurse's plan to move the patient slowly back into the community. Specif-ically, several women with whom the patient had a close relationship and with whom she rode to church were identified and elicited to begin taking her to church again. After several unsuccessful attempts, the patient began going to church again and at the time of termination was also going to lunch and to the local mall after church.

This was a drastic change of behavior on the part of the patient. Initially, she was cut off from most social contact except for her family and talked con-sistently about waiting to die. The final sign that Mrs. M. had regained some of her previous mental status was evident when she started to insist that she get her hair done at the local beauty salon. The fact that Mrs. M. began to be concerned about her personal appearance was evidence that her depression was improved, which made her more compliant with her diabetes and hy-pertension regime. Ongoing work with the family was focused on allowing the siblings to relinquish their care roles to the patient so that they could focus on their needs, such as employment, substance abuse treatment, and establishing independent lives.

A multisystem approach to urban poor families is the most therapeutic way to intervene with an identified patient with multiple problems such as di-abetes, hypertension, congestive heart failure, and depression. A compre-hensive focus that includes the health needs, the family structure and dynamics, family resources, and community resources must be considered in planning care for the patient. This case study demonstrates how nurses who are working in communities with African American, urban, poor families must explore and integrate into the care planning all resources and services that can be utilized to help the patient and family to restructure and change the family problem solving relative to the management of the patient's health and other family problems.

─────────ANNOTATED REFERENCES─────────

Aponte, H. J. (1994). *Bread and spirit: Therapy with the new poor: Diversity of race, culture, and values.* New York: Norton.

Harry Aponte has a long rich history of doing family therapy with poor disorganized African American and Latino families. This book contains his knowledge, beliefs, and values about how to best work with poor families from diverse racial, ethnic and cultural backgrounds. He demonstrates a holistic understanding of how societal and institutional norms and values influence all segments of a community. He advocates for training programs that will enhance awareness in therapist about how race, ethnicity, culture and socioeconomic status influence the patient, the therapist, and therefore therapy. With increased awareness of the therapist about race, ethnicity, and culture, he believes that the therapist will have more respect for the struggles, strengths, and the spirit of the poor and culturally diverse families that they are treating.

Boyd-Franklin, N. (1989). *Black families in therapy: A multisystems approach.* New York: Guilford Press.

This text, while out-of-date, is essential reading for anyone in healthcare who works with African American families. It is written to provide basic and advanced information to be used by practitioners at all levels. Dr. Boyd-Franklin has provided a comprehensive text about the history, theory, and clinical implications relative to the treatment of African American families. She tackles all the complex issues about African American people in this country such as examining how African American people in this country have distinct cultural and racial experiences but yet form diverse groups. Most importantly, in this text she offers clear guidance for joining, assessing and problem solving with African American families around health issues. These guidelines can be adapted by nurses in all types of practice.

McGoldrick, M., Giordano, J., & Pearce, J. (Eds.). (1996). *Ethnicity and family therapy* (2nd ed.). New York: Guilford Press.

The authors have revised their original publication on race, ethnicity, culture, and family therapy that was the first resource on culture, race, and ethnicity in the field of family therapy. The overview defines the concepts of ethnicity and the many factors relevant to ethnicity and family therapy history. Over twenty-three ethnic groups are discussed including their histories, migratory patterns, differences among the groups, and other pertinent facts. Implications for mental health treatment are suggested for each group.

Wilson, W. J. (1996) *When work disappears: The world of the new urban poor.* New York: Alfred A. Knopf.

William Julius Wilson has done seminal sociological work of the conditions of poor, urban African American people. In this latest work, he explains how inner-city residents have been impacted negatively by the loss of blue collar jobs in their community. He has developed a comprehensive analysis about how the effects of job loss in urban black communities isolate the poor. He also discusses the way in which potential employers view the urban poor and further isolate them by not offering them employment.

What is most important about Wilson's current work is his dismantling of the often-held premise that poor, urban black people lack motivation to work and achieve. Rather, he demonstrates through data analysis that the urban poor have the same aspirations for their lives and the lives of their children as the middle class. He explains the barriers that prevent them from obtaining the fulfillment of their goals. Finally, he offers public policy solutions to eradicate some of these problems. This book provides a framework by which practitioners can form, or in many cases, reform their own beliefs about the urban poor racially diverse groups that they serve.

Illuminating an Elderly Woman's Life

―――――――――――――――OBJECTIVES――――――――――――――

1. Describe how beliefs about rootwork, spells, and hexes among selected African Americans may influence their health attitudes, efficacy beliefs, and compliance with healthcare regimes.
2. Discuss how, among women of color, storytelling can be used as an effective method for learning more about their cultural beliefs about health problems and experiences.
3. Describe how the techniques of positive self-attributions and cognitive restructuring can be used to assist the patient with coping and complying better with healthcare plans by intervening in their dysfunctional beliefs and thought patterns related to the unnatural origin and progression of their health problems.

*M*rs. S. is a 90-year-old African American woman who looks at least ten years younger than her biological age. She is very tall and stately with very smooth, wrinkle-free, honey-brown skin. She has severe arthritis and congestive heart failure as well as other systems problems related to aging.

Mrs. S. was refereed to the psychiatric nurse, Visiting Nurse Association, because she was not consistently taking her prescribed medications. She believed that medications were not necessarily going to help her because her health problems were a direct result of a "spell" or "hex" that had been put on her by her mother-in-law many years ago. Mrs. S. believes that the aches and pains that she feels in her legs and her husband's sexual impotency are the result of the "spell." Therefore, she has felt powerless and hopeless about her situation.

She lives in a row house in a neighborhood that has been well maintained. She and her husband own their home in which they raised their three children. The children are all well-adjusted, productive adults who live in Philadelphia. Her children visit frequently and maintain a supportive relationship with their parents.

Mrs. S. and her husband married when she was 21 and he was 17 although she did not know he was younger than she until after they were married. She describes her husband's mother as being very possessive of her son and attributed her behavior to his age at the time of the marriage. Mr. S. has always worked hard to support his family and has been loyal over the years to his wife. Presently, he is the primary caretaker for her. Mrs. S. describes how her husband attends her in the middle of the night when she cannot make it to the bathroom, and changes her. She states that they have always "stuck together." She shared that, throughout the marriage, Mr. S. has been very apologetic to her about the way that his mother and grandmother treated her. He also believes that his mother and grandmother cast a spell on Mrs. S.

According to Mrs. S., her mother-in-law cast the spell on her when Mrs. S. refused to live with her anymore. Shortly after they were married, the couple moved in with her mother-in-law to help the family with living expenses as Mr. S. had a very good job as a chef. However, the other family members did not contribute to the household expenses. Mrs. S. did not consider moving out of her mother-in-law's house until her mother-in-law began to interfere in her role as mother. She shared that her mother-in-law constantly undermined her as mother and wife. Because of this conflict, Mrs. S. decided that they would move. When her husband agreed with her, his mother cast the spell on Mrs. S.

She and her husband migrated to Philadelphia over six decades ago with their three children. They were always an upwardly mobile family even when they lived in the South during the Depression. Mr. S. has always been employed, having been trained at an early age as a chef. Mrs. S. shared that, when they lived in the South during the Depression, Mr. S. had to wear white uniforms to work. Because the uniform identified him as a black man with a profession, he had to have an escort to accompany him to and from work to avoid being beaten by jealous white men.

Mr. and Mrs. S. are financially comfortable, and they have family and community support systems in place. Over the course of their marriage, however, they both have been very affected by their belief that Mr. S.'s mother cast a spell on Mrs. S. many decades ago. This belief has been reinforced by older family members, such as Mr. S.'s aunt, who have predicted that the couple's sex life must have been dismal because of the spell since the mother-in-law was overheard to say that Mr. S. would never "be any good to his wife." This was interpreted by the couple and other family members to mean that he would not be able to function sexually. Since Mr. S. has had impotency problems throughout the marriage, Mrs. S. accepts his impotency as validation of the power of the spell. For this reason, they have never sought medical or psychiatric evaluation of this problem.

Presently, Mrs. S. has difficulty with mobility. Since her house has two floors, she has an electronic lift that she uses to go up and down the stairs. On most days, she remains upstairs. On these days, her husband prepares and serves her meals.

Finally, Mrs. S. worries about her husband who has had to assume much of the responsibility for her care. She also believes that he is sad because of the way his family has treated them over the years.

QUESTIONS

1. Initially, what guidelines need to be followed by the nurse to facilitate a nursing assessment that demonstrates cultural competence?
2. With a client like Mrs. S., what actions would the nurse who is culturally competent not take?
3. How can the use of storytelling or narrative in the treatment of women of color be used as an effective treatment strategy?
4. How can the nurse learn to use cultural beliefs as metaphorical communication about life experiences as a woman of color to promote cognitive reframing about problems that impact on their health?
5. What family resources can the nurse strengthen to enhance the family system and restructure how Mrs. S. complies with the prescribed health regime?

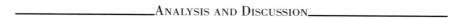

ANALYSIS AND DISCUSSION

This case study illuminates the life of a 90-year-old African American woman who has several chronic diseases that she attributes to her being placed under a spell by her mother-in-law many decades ago. Mrs. S. is the primary client although the family, especially her husband, had to be considered when planning healthcare interventions because he shares her belief about the origin of her sickness and his sexual dysfunction problems.

In this case, the primary function of the psychiatric nurse is to create an atmosphere of trust so that the patient is comfortable to share her thoughts and feelings about her physical and mental health. Family therapists such as Boyd-Franklin (1989) who work with African American families extensively believe that the person-to-person connection that the healthcare provider establishes with the patient is crucial. Without this personal connection, the patient will not view the healthcare provider as credible and, hence, will not be open to interventions suggested by the provider.

Because of her beliefs about the origin and inevitable outcome of her illness, Mrs. S. had frustrated her primary doctor and the visiting nurse who was assigned to her. The nurse described being unable to make any progress with the patient relative to having her comply with the care plan developed for her. The nurse also described the primary physician as being resigned to the fact that Mrs. S. would not follow the plan of treatment he had developed for her.

Being acutely aware of the need to foster a nurse-to-patient connection in the beginning, the psychiatric nurse consultant began the joining process with the patient by listening to the patient without judging or trying to refute her story about the origin of her illness. Additionally, the healthcare provider must use caution not to overreact when the patient's beliefs and values are different from the caregiver's. It is important that the nurse demonstrate a respect for the patient's beliefs and values by asking for clarification when needed while gathering information about the patient and her experiences. Much later in the process, the nurse can negotiate with the patient about beliefs and behaviors relative to her health regime. However, negotiation cannot take place before mutual respect between the patient and the nurse has been established. As suggested by Hines and Boyd-Franklin (1996), the healthcare provider has the greatest chance of being therapeutic when working within the confines of the family's and/or patient's belief system.

In this case, it meant that the nurse working with Mrs. S. had to listen to the patient express her beliefs about the origin of her illness without becoming overly fascinated with the exotic nature of the belief. Nor could the nurse refute Mrs. S.'s health beliefs. The function of the nurse was to listen to the patient, trying to understand the context of her beliefs as well as the meaning of the communication. Careful listening for the themes revealed that much of what the patient described had to do with the losses she had suffered over the years beginning with the loss of control over her own house and the parenting of her children when she moved in with her mother-in-law, whom she describes as usurping her authority in all of these areas. She was able to share that she had experienced long periods of depression that began during the early years of her marriage.

As the nurse continues to work with Mrs. S., she will need to include Mrs. S.'s husband in the sessions. They have a close relationship, sharing some of the same beliefs about the nature of the spell that was placed on them. Mrs. S. stated that she thought that her husband had experienced immense guilt and depression as a result of some of his mother's actions toward his family. The use of reminiscing with them as a couple in which they can review the challenges that they have met successfully, such as racism in the South and disruptive family members, they can also be encouraged to take credit as a couple for the parenting skills that they employed that produced successful, productive children who were loving and respectful of them.

With African American patients such as Mrs. S., cognitive restructuring is an approach that can be used effectively. Cognitive restructuring techniques are useful because they emphasize the practical that appeals to the cultural orientation of many African Americans. Using cognitive restructuring the nurse helped the patient to change negative thoughts by reframing them in a manner that encouraged positive thought patterns about her (and her husband's) ability to cope and problem-solve in very oppressive circumstances. For example, emphasis was placed on the love, respect, and strength they had as a couple that sustained them over the years under trying circumstances. Mr. S.'s continued devotion to her was highlighted as being a testimony to the love, respect, and loyalty in their marriage.

Mrs. S.'s case was complicated because a plan of care had to be developed that included interventions developed specifically for her physical well-being. However, barriers to the care plan had to be eradicated before the patient would agree to be compliant with the medical regime. The nurse had to gather data—in this case, in the form of a genogram—assess the family history, structure, strengths, and dynamics before interventions could be devised. Most importantly, the nurse, being culturally competent, used knowledge about how to work effectively with this African American elderly patient to achieve more positive health outcomes for the patient and her husband.

_____ANNOTATED REFERENCES_____

Capers, C. (Ed.). (1985). Cultural diversity and nursing practice. *Topics in Clinical Nursing, 7*(3).

This volume is over 10 years old but the seminal work found in all eleven articles is important content for nurses at all levels who work with diverse groups of patients. The volume contains a general overview of what nurses need to understand about culture and ethnicity when they work with diverse groups of patients. Following the overview, selected racially cultural diverse groups are discussed. Suggestions are made by the authors about how to deliver culturally competent care to the specific groups. Additionally, special topics such as the influences of religion on the health beliefs of African Americans and how to transcend cultural bias are discussed. The information in this volume is written in a clear and concise manner and much of the information is timeless.

Comas-Diez, B. & Green, B. (Eds.). (1994). *Women of color: Integrating ethnic and gender identities in psychotherapy.* New York: Guilford Press.

This book contains a comprehensive explanation of the mental health status of women of color. It provides guidelines for providing mental healthcare to women of color that is culturally competent and gender-sensitive. The book is organized around three working paradigms: Women of color: a portrait of heterogeneity which includes a historical overview; developmental issues, sociocultural issues, family issues, and gender issues; Part II—Applied Framework which explains the various theoretical models that have been effective with women of color, guidelines for their use are included; Part III—Special Populations of women of color and their unique needs are highlighted. Some of the groups discussed are professional women of color, lesbians, and mixed-race women. This book is comprehensive and extremely important. It provides copious information about women of color and their mental health needs. It is extensive and the guidelines provided for culturally competent care are excellent.

McAdoo, H. P. (Ed.). (1993). *Family ethnicity: A strength in diversity.* Newbury Park, CA: Sage.

Harriet McAdoo has a distinguished history writing and researching about ethnicity and family treatment. This edited volume is unique in that it looks at family-related issues that have to do with ethnicity instead of the typical ethnic focus which looks at individuals or groups as the frame of reference. McAdoo provides the theoretical framework for understanding the information presented in this volume. Demographics on selected ethnic groups are presented and issues of diversity such as social class and minority status are discussed. The reminder of the book contains chapters that provide extensive explanation of issues related to the major minority groups in this country. This volume contains a well thought out framework for understanding diversity and ethnicity among selected groups of people.

McGoldrick, M., Giordano, J., & Pearce, J. (Eds.). (1996). *Ethnicity and family therapy* (2nd ed.). New York: Guilford Press.

The authors have revised their original publication on race, ethnicity, culture, and family therapy that was the first resource on culture, race, and ethnicity in the field of family therapy. The overview defines the concepts of ethnicity and the many factors relevant to ethnicity and family therapy history. Over 23 ethnic groups are discussed including their histories, migratory patterns, differences among the groups, and other pertinent facts. Implications for mental health treatment are suggested for each group. The chapter developed by Hines and Boyd-Franklin was used extensively as a reference for this case study.

Chapter 4

A Perspective on Latino Healthcare

Antonia Villarruel, PhD, RN

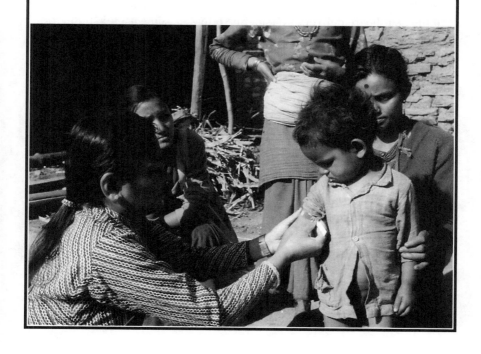

COMMENTARY

Vernice D. Ferguson

The Latino population in the United States is growing at a rapid rate. We can learn much from this community about cultural sensitivity based on their ability to pick up the cultural nuances of a given situation quickly. This ability has been observed in other minority groups as well. With it comes the desire to be treated with respect.

An article appeared in the *Washington Post* that addressed the rise of Latino executives on the corporate ladder and their business edge in international markets (Aguilar, 1996). Hector Ruiz, an executive vice president and general manager for Motorola Inc., oversees worldwide markets of Motorola's paging business. He stated, "We deal with two cultures all our lives, integrating them into our own; I've seen it translate into a natural business edge for Latinos. It means you're often able to absorb the cultural differences of a new market and the changing workforce. And if people can sense you respect them and you catch on quickly, they want to work with you."

In healthcare, our goal is to empower people to take charge of their lives effectively. Dr. Villarruel provides us with three scenarios to assist us in identifying cultural and structural barriers that Latinos face in the healthcare delivery system. She offers us some useful strategies to minimize these barriers while helping us to recognize some of the important cultural values as the Latino population is served.

Aguilar, L. For Latino executives, a profitable perspective. *Washington Post*. September 8, 1996.

Health Promotion Strategies

1. Identify strategies in designing successful health promotion programs in the Latino community.
2. Recognize the benefits and limitations of adapting health promotion strategies developed for majority populations for culturally diverse populations.

*M*s. W. is employed by a large university medical center. She has been assigned the task of writing a proposal for the purpose of establishing a community-based bilingual birthing class for the Latino community. Ms. W. is planning to translate an existing curriculum that is being used at the medical center because she believes it has been effective. Further, there are limited funds available to develop a specific curriculum for Latinos. She plans to conduct most of the programs herself. Although she is not bilingual, she is counting on having one of the agency staff available to translate. However, the grant is not sufficient to cover the cost of the translator. Ms. W. develops the proposal and, prior to submission, contacts the local Latino community health center for their support. In addition to providing a translator, Ms. W. requests that the community health center identify potential program participants. Ms. W. is surprised by the resistance on the part of the center's administration for what she perceives as a program that would assist the 500 prenatal women who enroll in the clinic. The center director tells Ms. W. that the program will not work in the community as designed. Ms. W. is perplexed because the model has been successful at the Medical Center.

QUESTIONS

1. What strategies should have been used by Ms. W. in designing the program?

2. What are some reasons that the program as designed by Ms. W. would not work in the community health center?
3. What elements would you include in order to make the program a success?

ANALYSIS AND DISCUSSION

What constitutes a culturally appropriate intervention? Providing relevant information in the language of the target population is an important element. However, translation alone is *not sufficient* to ensure health information will be received in a useful manner by the target population. Other important elements in designing culturally appropriate interventions include: (a) basing the intervention on the cultural values of the targeted group; (b) making the intervention accessible by considering at minimal the cost, time, and location involved with the information or intervention; and (c) ensuring that strategies which comprise the intervention reflect the attitudes, expectancies, and norms of the target population regarding a particular behavior (Marin, 1993).

The approach that Ms. W. took in this situation—utilizing an approach that has been successful with one cultural group and using it with another— is very common. Often, health promotion strategies are developed for the majority culture and because of time and cost constraints, minimal adaptations are made when the intervention is utilized with diverse groups of people. The limitations of this approach, as seen in this case study, concern interventions that may not be viewed by the targeted communities as necessary or effective.

Without any community consultation, Ms. W. made the assumption that birthing classes were necessary. She further assumed that the classroom format would be an effective means of providing this information, and that despite her inability to speak Spanish she would be an appropriate person to teach the classes. Ms. W. did not explore community concerns related to childbirth, nor did she evaluate the strengths, resources, or means of communication that might be preferred in designing this program.

Questions Ms. W. might have considered in bringing this program to the clinic include: What information do women and their families want and need to have? Who should participate in these classes? What barriers might there be to women participating in a series of classes? Who is the most credible person to deliver this information? Is it a health provider or perhaps another member of the community or health center?

The lack of consultation with the community is especially problematic since the community health clinic is being asked to assume major time and responsibility for the program. The reactions and resistance by persons in the community health clinic to the approach used by Ms. W. are understandable. The development of culturally sensitive and effective strategies is a time-intensive effort. However, a true collaborative relationship can facilitate the development, effectiveness, and sustainability of health promotion strategies.

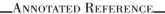
ANNOTATED REFERENCE

Marin, G. (1993). Defining culturally appropriate community interventions: Hispanics as a case study. *Journal of Community Psychology, 21,* 149–161.

This article establishes the importance and rationale for the development of community wide behavior change interventions directed at behavior change that are group specific and culturally appropriate. Using Hispanics as a case study, components of culturally appropriate interventions are defined.

Enhancing Preventive Care

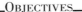

OBJECTIVES

1. Identify cultural and structural barriers to preventive care faced by Latinas.
2. Discuss strategies to minimize barriers to preventive care for Latinas.

A Comprehensive Cancer Center is considering conducting a Cancer Education and Screening Program for Latina women. Currently, city and county monies are available for breast and cervical cancer screening; however there has been a low rate of participation among Latina women. As the program is currently designed, women are screened for eligibility to participate in the screening at a local community health center. If they are determined to be eligible, another appointment is made for them at the local health department which is 10 miles away from the neighborhood. While women have participated in the eligibility screening, there has been a low rate of follow-up for the screening mammogram and pap smear. The health department has contacted the Comprehensive Cancer Center to assist in addressing the problem that has been determined to have resulted from a lack of education about cancer.

A beginning needs assessment has identified the following problems: (a) although a relatively short distance from the community to the health center, it takes two bus transfers and approximately 3 hours for women to reach the local health department; (b) there are no bilingual personnel at the local health department; (c) several women have reported that local health department staff have treated people rudely and have yelled at them for not speaking English; (d) women fear that if they are found to have cancer, they won't be able to seek treatment because they have limited insurance; (e) although many of the women are legal residents, several women reported that the staff at the health department stated these services are "for Americans only."

---QUESTIONS---

1. As a nurse at the Comprehensive Cancer Center, how would you begin to design the Cancer Awareness Program?
2. What other factors might you need to address?
3. Who would you enlist to assist you in the design and implementation of the program?

---ANALYSIS AND DISCUSSION---

Transportation, lack of bilingual personnel, perceived discrimination, lack of insurance, and anti-immigrant sentiment are some of the structural barriers confronted by Latinos in seeking primary and secondary healthcare. In research studies, each of these barriers has been associated with limited use of healthcare services among Latinos. Thus is it important that these barriers be addressed in the design of healthcare services for Latino populations. While the health department perceived women in the Latina community as having a lack of education about breast and cervical cancer, the needs assessment conducted identified many structural barriers. Several strategies can be used to minimize these barriers to screening services.

First, it would be important to build on the partnership with the local community health center. To the extent possible, services should be available within the neighborhood in conjunction with the local community health center. Such a partnership would minimize the need for additional transportation to a location that is perceived by community members as not receptive to Latinos. If services need to be obtained at the health department or the Comprehensive Cancer Center, accommodations for monolingual Spanish-speaking persons will need to be made. Again, an effective community partnership would be instrumental in developing options for effective translator services. The need for cultural competence training to facilitate working with Latino populations should also be determined.

Another strategy to decrease barriers or the perception of barriers by Latina women involves the design of information about the program. It would be important to incorporate some of the concerns identified in the needs assessment, such as, How much will this cost me? What if I don't have insurance? What happens if I have an abnormal finding? Do I have to be a citizen in order to receive treatment? Further, credible means of disseminating information and preferred formats for receiving information should also be identified. Conducting a focus group or interviewing users of screening services would be an important means of gathering information in the development of effective cancer screening programs.

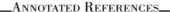

_____ANNOTATED REFERENCES_____

Giachello, A. (1994). Issues of access and use. In C. W. Molina & M. Aguirre-Molina (Eds.) *Latino health in the U.S.: A growing challenge* (pp. 63–111). Washington, DC: APHA.

This chapter provides a comprehensive synthesis of theory and research related to issues of health access and use among Latino populations. Traditional barriers including regular sources of care, health insurance and other barriers are discussed. Specific issues related to special populations including undocumented workers, migrant/seasonal workers, and Puerto Ricans who travel back and forth to the mainland are also presented.

Surgeon General's National Workshop on Hispanic Latino/Health. (1982). *Blueprint for improving Hispanic/Latino health: Implementation strategies* [Workshop Proceedings] Washington, DC: Office of the Surgeon General.

These proceedings are a summary of key issues and recommendations from national and regional meetings of the Surgeon General's Hispanic/Latino Health Initiative. Priority areas of this landmark initiative included findings and recommendations to: (a) improve access to healthcare; (b) improve data collection strategies; (c) develop a relevant and comprehensive research agenda; (d) increase representation in the science and health professions; and (e) improve health promotion and disease prevention.

Understanding the Role of
Cultural Norms

1. Define the cultural values of familialism, respeto, and prescribed gender roles.
2. Recognize the importance the cultural values of familialism, respeto, and prescribed gender roles when dealing with Latino families.

*L*inda G. is a 15-year-old Mexican-American who has been an A student. Her teacher notices she has been missing a great deal of school. When she is in school, she is extremely tired. As a school nurse, you have been requested to make a home visit. Upon visiting her home, you meet her father Juan G., a 37-year-old Mexican-American male. Mr. G. was injured at work, having fallen from a ladder. The job was an "under-the-table" incident and he has been unable to collect disability or unemployment. He is suffering from chronic back pain and is unable to work. Mr. G. does not want to take pain killers because he is afraid of becoming addicted. He takes and uses a number of different remedies that friends have given him from Mexico. In addition, he has sought treatment from homeopaths and other physicians in Mexico. Beatrice G., his wife, has begun to work full-time since the accident in order to pay medical bills and support the family. Mr. G. indicates that he needs Linda at home to cook for the family and to help him take care of the three younger children. He believes that Linda will probably get married in a few years, so it is not as important at this time for her to attend school. He has made an effort to do some things around the house, but at times he is physically unable. He indicates that he no longer has any friends and states he feels many neighbors talk about him because he is the "woman of the house." Although pleasant, Mr. G. states that the situation is a family matter and no one from the school should be telling him how to run his family. After talking to Linda, you notice some signs of depression. She likes going to school and has dreams of going to college to become a nurse.

1. What approach would you use in working with Mr. G.?
2. What approach would you use in working with Linda?
3. What are potential conflicts in the approach you choose or consider?

ANALYSIS AND DISCUSSION

In working with the family, the cultural factors of respeto, familialism, and prescribed gender roles are critical to consider. Respeto, or respect, dictates the appropriate differential behavior toward others on the basis of age, socioeconomic position, gender, and authority status. The concept of familialism refers to reciprocal relationships of responsibility, loyalty, and support among family and extended family members. Finally, within Latino culture there is a traditional prescription of roles that is determined by gender. For example, women are viewed as having major caretaking responsibilities within the home, while men have responsibilities for providing for the family.

At a minimum the nurse in this situation needs to: (a) show respect for cultural values and practices held by Mr. G. and his family; (b) acknowledge those beliefs and values as important; and (c) attempt to find solutions or options within the cultural framework. Thus, the nurse must be careful to see that her feelings about Linda and her situation do not interfere with the families decisions in this situation.

An important strategy here would involve the nurse in working with and earning the respect of Mr. G. His position within the family and responsibility as decision-maker for the entire family needs to be acknowledged. His position as head of the family might currently be threatened because of his inability to provide economically for his family. Efforts of the nurse then might be directed at Mr. G. so as to obtain adequate pain relief. Addressing his concern about addiction as well as incorporating effective and safe alternative remedies should be considered. Identifying resources within the community for job training, and assistance with medical insurance would be important in addressing some of his concerns. In addition, identifying family members to provide assistance with responsibilities around the home and with the younger children might relieve Linda of some of these responsibilities.

It would be important to support Linda during this time. Identifying family members to provide assistance with the care of the home and younger children might relieve Linda of some of these responsibilities. Providing encouragement and praise for her support of her family and her work at home should be provided.

_____REFERENCES_____

Marin, G., & Marin, B. V. (1991). *Research with Hispanic populations.* Newbury Park, CA: Sage.

Molina, C., Zambrana, R. E., & Aguirre-Molina, M. (1994). In C. W. Molina & M. Aguirre-Molina (Eds.) *Latino health in the U.S.: A growing challenge* (pp. 23–43). Washington, DC: APHA.

_____ANNOTATED REFERENCES_____

Giachello, A. (1994). Issues of access and use. In C. W. Molina & M. Aguirre-Molina (Eds.), *Latino health in the U.S.: A growing challenge* (pp. 63–111). Washington, DC: APHA.

This chapter provides a comprehensive synthesis of theory and research related to issues of health access and use among Latino populations. Traditional barriers including regular sources of care, health insurance and other barriers are discussed. Specific issues related to special populations including undocumented workers, migrant/seasonal workers, and Puerto Ricans who travel back and forth to the mainland are also presented.

Marin, G. (1993). Defining culturally appropriate community interventions: Hispanics as a case study. *Journal of Community Psychology, 21,* 149–161.

This article establishes the importance and rationale for the development of community wide behavior change interventions directed at behavior change that are group specific and culturally appropriate. Using Hispanics as a case study, components of culturally appropriate interventions are defined.

Molina, C., Zambrana, R. E., & Aguirre-Molina, M. (1994). The influence of culture, class, and environment on health care. In C. W. Molina & M. Aguirre-Molina (Eds.), *Latino health in the U.S.: A growing challenge* (pp. 23–43). Washington, DC: APHA.

This chapter provides a theoretical perspective. An overview of "traditional" Latino values as well as beliefs and practices related to health and illness are presented.

Surgeon General's National Workshop on Hispanic Latino/Health. (1982). *Blueprint for improving Hispanic/Latino health: Implementation strategies* [Workshop Proceedings] Washington, DC: Office of the Surgeon General.

These proceedings are a summary of key issues and recommendations from national and regional meetings of the Surgeon General's Hispanic/Latino Health Initiative. Priority areas of this landmark initiative included findings and recommendations to: (a) improve access to healthcare; (b) improve data collection strategies; (c) develop a relevant and comprehensive research agenda; (d) increase representation in the science and health professions; and (e) improve health promotion and disease prevention.

Villarruel, A. M. (1995). Mexican-American cultural meanings, expressions, self-care, and dependent-care actions associated with pain. *Research in Nursing and Health, 18,* 427–436.

The purpose of this ethnographic study was to discover Mexican-American meanings, expressions, and care associated with pain. Based on study findings, a beginning description of the cultural context is provided from which pain as experienced by Mexican-Americans can be understood and from which culturally competent nursing care can be designed.

Chapter 5

HIGH-RISK CARE IN URBAN AMERICA

Katherine K. Kinsey

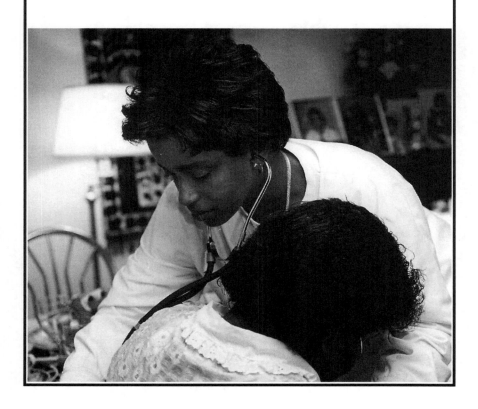

COMMENTARY

Vernice D. Ferguson

Many African-American families are at high risk in urban America. In these case studies, Dr. Kinsey reminds us that responding to an individual in need of nursing care is short-sighted unless attention is paid to the individual's family structure, its dynamics and the impact of the surrounding community. The extended family and often the intergenerational conflict which surfaces must be understood if nursing care is to be effective. Students soon learn that providing nursing services in the community is quite complex and demands much more of them compared to what they have learned to provide in a more controlled and predictable setting such as the hospital.

The Influence of Family Dynamics

--------------------OBJECTIVES--------------------

1. Describe four or more barriers to optimal family healthcare.
2. Develop three or more strategies to engage client/family in plan of care.
3. Discuss the influence of cultural, community and environmental factors on individual and family health indices.

*M*s. L. is a 22-year-old African-American woman enrolled in a Perinatal Home Visiting Program (PHVP). She enrolled in the program when she was 7 months pregnant with her fourth child. Ms. L. delayed prenatal care until her second trimester since she moved from one neighborhood to another "to get away from my mother." She delivered a low birth-weight infant (5 pounds) two weeks before her due date. Within the first month of life, her son James was diagnosed with esophageal reflux and failure to thrive.

Ms. L. also has two daughters, age 7 and 2 years. She lost a son (7 months old) to Sudden Infant Death Syndrome (SIDS) four years ago. Soon after his death, she became pregnant with her second daughter. This child was born prematurely at 35 weeks. Nine months later, Ms. L. became pregnant with James. These two short interval pregnancies resulted in low birth-weight newborns. Each newborn remained in the Neonatal Intensive Care Unit for 7 days.

After hospital discharge, Ms. L. and James had weekly (or more often as indicated) home visits by the Public Health Nurse of the Perinatal Home Visiting Program. In addition, the pediatric staff at the local university hospital evaluated James on a monthly basis. By four months, James began to gain weight and stabilize. The day after his last pediatric appointment, Ms. L. found James dead in the crib. The diagnosis was SIDS.

Three months after his death, Ms. L. openly expresses her grief about her two losses. "Why did my sons die?" She says her family is "sick and tired of her problems and crying." She reports that she is smoking more now than ever before (2 to 3 packs of cigarettes/day). And her current boyfriend tells her that it is important to have another baby "real quick" so she can "feel better."

Ms. L. lives with her 55-year-old grandmother (Mrs. S.). The grandmother is the informal custodian of five of the seven children of Ms. L.'s mother. Ms. L.'s mother, who is homeless and HIV+, has been a crack addict since 1986. She openly abandoned her minor children two years ago and Mrs. S. assumed parenting responsibilities.

The household composition is:

Grandmother (age 55): Mrs. S.
Grandchildren
   Adult Grandchild: Ms. L. (age 22)
      Great-granddaughter (age 7)
      Great-granddaughter (age 2)
Minor Grandchildren:
   Granddaughter (age 14)
   Grandson: (age 13)
   Granddaughter (age 10)
   Grandson (age 9)
   Granddaughter (age 4)
Grandson's girlfriend (age 19) This grandson is incarcerated for armed robbery in a federal penitentiary.
   Great-grandson (age 1)

The multigenerational family lives in a row home situated in a city block with several abandoned homes. The corner house is known as the neighborhood "crack" house. Last year, the house next door was torched by warring drug gangs. Graffiti covers many of the homes and fences. Ms. L. complains about the graffiti but says "There's 'nothin' we can do to stop it." Within the last month, two murders and one rape occurred in the immediate neighborhood. Drive-by shootings are not uncommon incidents.

Ms. L. dropped out of school in ninth grade; however, her younger brothers and sisters in the household are enrolled in school (but not doing well). Ms. L. has never been employed outside the home and she lacks job skills. She has been a recipient of public assistance since her eldest child, now age 7, was born.

Ms. L.'s current boyfriend (the father of James) has a history of substance abuse (heroin) and is not employed. Ms. L. states there are times when he has threatened her and "shoved me around." Then "he gets real sorry and says he'll never do that again." Since James died, three months ago, Ms. L. has had three pregnancy tests. The first two were negative. The third was positive. This is the third short-interval pregnancy for Ms. L. She is now in the process of deciding on a prenatal care provider.

During the Public Health Nurse visits, Ms. L.'s grandmother is always present. The grandmother participates in the discussions and frequently offers her opinions about what Ms. L. has done wrong in her life and how she should not be pregnant "again." "You should be moving out of my house . . . not having more babies. Why doesn't your boyfriend take you in since he wants you to have this baby so much?" "I have enough worries of my own with all these other kids and how they aren't doing well in school. I have other stuff bothering me, too. I sure don't need anymore."

QUESTIONS

1. As a public health nurse, what are three or more critical healthcare, social, and educational needs of Ms. S.?
2. What are barriers to optimal family healthcare as highlighted in this case study?
3. What are two critical environmental/community characteristics that influence access to healthcare?
4. What is one characteristic of this extended family that reflects this minority group's cultural norms and values?

ANALYSIS AND DISCUSSION

This case study presents the challenges of individuals and extended families living in a culturally diverse urban setting. Ms. L., as the primary client, has a variety of health, social, and educational needs. In addition, the family dynamics influence her health status as well as critical parenting roles and responsibilities.

As the Public Health Nurse (PHN) develops a plan of care, she or he must involve Ms. L. as a partner in decision-making processes. Mutual work regarding life goals, current and future family needs, and workable strategies is critical. If the PHN and the client do not understand the assumptions and priorities of each, there is little room to negotiate about goals and less opportunity to achieve goals. For example, sustaining the health of Ms. L. during this pregnancy as well as extending the pregnancy to term will be critical concerns of the Public Health Nurse. Although it might seem as critical to Ms. L. since she tells the nurse she wants this baby, the more important matter to her might be to learn more about SIDS: understanding the client's perspective strengthens the ultimate design of the care plan. The final care plan should incorporate timelines for prenatal appointments and regularly scheduled home visits. Other areas of work include strategies for smoking control/cessation, parenting and childbirth education, and the development of productive relationships with extended family members.

The public health nurse is responsible for developing and nurturing communication techniques which invite constructive input by family members and significant others. Educational sessions over time regarding mother-child care and family development during home visits by the PHN will facilitate client-nurse-family dialogue. Such one-on-one and small group sessions further support skill development in successful parenting. One essential approach to case management is acknowledging the challenges of urban life. The client and her family witness or experience personal and community threats regularly. Their economic resources are limited; they are not able to leave this environment. The public health nurse can strategize with the client as well as community members about this threatening environment (i.e., abandoned homes, crack houses, high crime neighborhoods). In addition, the public health nurse should practice community advocacy work. Frequently, clients living in high stress environmental conditions have had little experience affecting positive community changes. Due to social isolation, frequent moves and finite economics, clients lack the skills to identify and work closely with elected officials, merchants, and neighbors to improve their community. The public health nurse can develop and strengthen advocacy roles regarding housing, crime and violence for self and client(s).

It is important to recognize and value the culturally-derived support system in place, which is a valuable resource for Ms. L. The role of informal caregiver assumed by the grandmother (after raising six children of her own) demonstrates the cultural values and experiences of the African American family. It is not atypical for extended family members to assume parenting roles for children in time of crises. It is less likely that African American children will be placed for adoption or into formal foster care situations. The valuing of kinship and rearing of children is demonstrated by this family constellation. This structure and cultural feature should be respected by the public health nurse and viewed as a positive characteristic of the family. And the PHN should be attentive to Mrs. S.'s comments; her expressed frustration with her granddaughter's current situation does not translate into evicting her from the home.

Other features of this case must be incorporated into the service plan. Ms. L. needs much support as she continues with this pregnancy. Despite the number of children she has had, she is a young 22-year-old mother who started her family at the age of 15. In addition, her education is incomplete. She finished the ninth grade but has not returned for GED study. She has never worked outside the home. Education and job skills are critical goals to establish with Ms. L. The work to support realistic goals will be challenging and ongoing. In this regard, it may be more pragmatic to work with Ms. L. about short-term goals that she can successfully achieve regarding school and work. Long-range goals that consume more resources and time should be gradually introduced into the plan of care.

Ms. L's relationship with the father of her unborn appears tenuous. Issues of domestic violence and abuse must be carefully and skillfully addressed by the public health nurse. In addition, the public health nurse should identify other resources available in the community to work with Ms. L. regarding personal safety and family security. Sharing these resources and facilitating work with support organizations by Ms. S. will be the responsibility of the public health nurse.

Although Ms. L. is the principal client, family life and needs will influence how she plans and works to take care of herself and others. The context of family life is critical to consider and to incorporate into the plan of care. For example, the grandmother reports that the other children are having problems in school. Frequent moves and changing family structure may influence school performance and behavior. The needs of the children in the household may require other services in the home, school, and community. The public health nurse can be one resource to the family and can be a pivotal professional in initiating and following up on referrals not only for the minor children but for Ms. L. also.

Although the needs of Ms. L. seem quite obvious from this case study, much must be considered when developing an appropriate, mutually acceptable plan of care. The health, social, and educational history of the client must be reviewed; the current physical, mental, and emotional well-being of the client must be considered. In addition, family structure, dynamics, and community life are essential elements in developing the plan of care. Other elements include the physical and cultural environment of the community of residence. If the plan of care incorporates the contextual components of the case study, the opportunities for positive, healthy client and family outcomes expand.

—————————————ANNOTATED REFERENCES—————————————

Baldwin, K., & Chen, S. (1996). Use of public health nursing services: Relationship to adequacy of prenatal care and infant outcome. *Public Health Nursing, 13*(1), 13–20.

This article discusses a study of relationships among public health nursing contacts to downstate Illinois childbearing women, the adequacy of their prenatal medical care, and infant birthweight and gestational age outcomes. The authors found that the timing of initial public health nursing contact was significantly correlated with the adequacy of prenatal physician contact and infant gestational age. Early casefinding to identify and engage pregnant women in public health nursing and prenatal medical services is supported.

Beck-Sague, C., & Morese, S. (1996). Commentary on preterm births: Prevention of prematurity in black and white. *Public Health Reports, 3*, 114–115.

This brief commentary speaks to the study published in the March/April 1996 issue of *Public Health Reports* on "Racial disparities in preterm births: The role of urogenital infections." Author K. Fiscella. Beck-Sague and Morese advocate for continuing efforts to identify and address medical, social, cultural, and other factors that may affect the risk of preterm birth. The authors stress the need to provide available, accessible quality prenatal care to underserved populations, particularly low-income African American women.

Cameron, R., Wells, J., & Hbofoll, S. (1996). Stress, social support, and coping in pregnancy. *Journal of Health Psychology, 1*(2), 195–208.

Cameron and Wells examine data from two studies of pregnant women's coping with increased role demands in the context of current social support literature. They recognize current limitations in the social support literature to fully address the social realities of women of diverse racial backgrounds and socioeconomic conditions. The authors propose a new model of coping by pregnant women that is prosocial, active, and effective.

Dimperiro, D., Adams, C., Hale, C., Sierra, T., & Millsaps, C. (1996). Reducing the impact of substance abuse for at-risk women and infants. *Journal of Wellness Perspectives, 12*(2), 90–97.

The authors describe the initial findings of a federally funded demonstration project utilizing community-based preventive and preconceptional health promotion strategies targeting substance abusing women. The subjects resided in a rural area that is limited in its health and social service resources. Preliminary data suggest that clients benefited from project services and that utilizing paraprofessional home visitors with at-risk women and their infants is a promising strategy.

Gelles, J. (1996, March 28). New studies paint a vivid picture of the homeless in Philadelphia. *Philadelphia Inquirer*, A1, A20.

This newspaper article presents various findings regarding the homeless in an urban setting. Gelles uses the information to vividly portray the characteristics of those who have no permanent residence and to debunk the commonly held perception that the majority of homeless are older adult substance abusing minority males. In this east coast city, single women and their children or two-parent families are more apt to be those who seek shelter.

Lieberman, E. (1995). Low birth weight—not a black-and-white issue [Editorial]. *New England Journal of Medicine, 332*(2), 117–118.

This editorial presents the position that alternative approaches be explored to clarify reasons for the disparity in pregnancy outcomes between races. Lieberman uses the article by Rawlings et al. in this issue of the *Journal* to develop this perspective and urges future work to elucidate the reasons for excess rate of low birthweight infants born to African American women in America.

McDuffie, R., Beck, A., Bischoof, K., Cross, J., & Orleans, M. (1996). Effect of frequency of prenatal care visits on perinatal outcome among low-risk women. *Journal of the American Medical Association, 275*(11), 847–851.

Findings of a randomized controlled trial that involved low-risk pregnant women enrolled in a group model health maintenance organization are analyzed. Outcome measures including preterm delivery, cesarean delivery, low birthweight, and satisfaction with care were examined. Data documented that good perinatal outcomes and patient satisfaction were maintained when low-risk women adhered to the Public Health Service Expert Panel schedule of prenatal care (minimum of nine visits).

Wood, D., Halfon, N., Scarlata, D., Newacheck, P., & Nessim, S. (1993). Impact of family relocation on children's growth, development, school function and behavior. *Journal of the American Medical Association, 270*(11), 1334–1338.

The authors examine the influences of societal mobility and family relocation on approximately 10,000 American children. Parents reported their children's delays in growth or development, learning disorders, school failure, and frequent behavioral problems. It was found that frequent family relocation was associated with an increased risk of children failing a grade in school or four or more recurring behavioral problems.

An Intergenerational Family

—————————————OBJECTIVES—————————————

1. Describe four or more cultural influences on healthcare decisions by minority population.
2. Identify three or more health and social resources available to client.
3. Develop three or more strategies to engage client in plan of care.

*M*rs. S. is a 55-year-old African American woman who has lived in a quiet Philadelphia neighborhood for 35 years. She and her common-law husband moved here from Atlanta, Georgia, in 1960 to find better work. Her husband died in 1974 and she was left with six young children to raise. She and her family received AID to Families with Dependent Children (AFDC) and other public funds until her youngest child was 18. Three daughters live nearby and have growing families of their own. Two sons and the fourth daughter are heavy into drugs. The two sons are heroin addicts; the daughter has been addicted to crack cocaine since the mid-1980s.

The quiet neighborhood where Mrs. S. owns her home has changed in the past six years. Homes in adjacent blocks were condemned by the city due to ground settlement. Homes are abandoned by owners; drug dealers and squatters stay in the abandoned homes. Graffiti is painted on many of the homes and businesses. The nearby school has a known "crack" house across the block.

Mrs. S. never finished high school but finally started a GED program at age 53 when her addicted daughter's neglect of her grandchildren forced Mrs. S. to make a decision. She decided to take her "grandbabies" in (because she couldn't bear to know they were in foster homes or find out they were in a homeless shelter again). She dropped out of the GED program.

Mrs. S. is not proud of the fact that her grandson has been convicted of a federal offense and is incarcerated. But she felt she had to take in his girlfriend and their young child otherwise they too would have been homeless. (See case, "The Influence of Family Dynamics," p. 61.)

Mrs. S. finally felt she was getting her younger grandchildren's lives together when Ms. L. (the oldest granddaughter) showed up on the door step with her two children and pregnant again. Now there are " . . . 11 people in the house . . . I never thought I would be taking care of so many people again."

Mrs. S. expresses frustration with her circumstances and shares her concern about the grandchildren who are growing up without a mother. The only time they see their mother is when she shows up to beg for drug money.

Mrs. S. is upset about her youngest grandson dying of SIDS in her home. She thinks it must have something to do with her granddaughter's smoking "so much." She is worried about Ms. L.'s current pregnancy and what might happen again. She also frets about housing and wishes Ms. L. could be on her own and live independently.

In addition, Mrs. S. reports that she has not seen her doctor in two years. "I'm too busy worrying about these kids and how they are doing in school besides my other granddaughter (age 14) got pregnant and we had to take care of her. But maybe I should go see someone. See, I think I have this lump in my breast. My sister died of breast cancer four years ago and I have never forgotten how awful that was. Maybe this is just a cyst. I think I will pray on it and wait a little longer to see if it goes away. If it goes away, that means I don't have to worry about that right now. But you know I know three of my church friends have breast cancer and they all live around here. Maybe it's something in the air. I sure hope it's nothing, 'cause I have gotta be around for the grandbabies."

_____QUESTIONS_____

1. How do you view your nursing responsibilities and relationship with Mrs. S.?
2. What are cultural barriers that could influence Mrs. S.'s decisions regarding the access and use of breast healthcare services?
3. What are three strategies the public health nurse could use to support Mrs. S. as she works through her issues regarding risk of breast cancer, the fear of a similar experience (like her sister), and the urgency to seek medical consultation?
4. What community characteristics could influence Mrs. S.'s use of primary care services for her personal health, particularly as it relates to breast health?

_____ANALYSIS AND DISCUSSION_____

Mrs. S. has not been the focus of care services by the public health nurse. Her 22-year-old granddaughter was identified through Outreach and eligible for free Perinatal Home Visiting Services. Over time the family constellation and dynamics became critical components in developing an appropriate plan of care with Ms. L. and Mrs. S.

Over time, Mrs. S. has been able to communicate with the public health nurse her experiences regarding parenting responsibilities of grandchildren, the changing neighborhood, the issues of personal health, and particular family experiences. The family history of breast cancer, the self-detection of a lump are significant factors when the public health nurse counsels Mrs. S. Counseling, referral, and follow-up are critical for Mrs. S. even if she has not been the principal client. The astute public health nurse should be sensitive to cultural interpretations regarding care of self and mortality. It will be critical to work with this "secondary" client also.

An accepting, proactive stance should be assumed by the public health nurse. Recriminations about doing something earlier would not be an acceptable position to take with Mrs. S. In addition, this punitive approach elicits guilt feelings and defensive behaviors on the part of the client. Such behaviors neither support optimal decision making about healthcare needs nor construct therapeutic relationships.

Another concern Mrs. S. might have is financial. She may worry about the moneys it takes for screening and subsequent medical treatment. In addition, she may be concerned more immediately with the ongoing care of many minor children. If she is sick, who will take care of them? The public health nurse must be familiar with community resources that could assist Mrs. S. in covering the cost of diagnosis and treatment. In addition, the issues of family custody and ongoing parenting responsibilities must be addressed along with concerns about community stability and ongoing threats to personal safety. The public health nurse must view the community as an entity that can influence health related decisions. For example, Mrs. S. may fear traveling to and from the local hospital and will avoid making or keeping necessary appointments. The PHN should incorporate into the plan of care a system of monitoring appointments and the barriers influencing the kept appointment rate.

As the public health nurse continues to work with Mrs. S. and Ms. L., financial issues should be examined repeatedly. Although household management and the worry about making it until the end of the month may not be expressed openly, they are sources of much apprehension. Clients should be referred to financial counseling services as indicated. In particular, if a critical health threat emerges, family dialogue should be initiated regarding economic concerns, household management, and community resources, such as the American Cancer Society.

The need to develop a care plan for Mrs. S. is evident. She has expressed primary healthcare and educational needs. Without guidance and support by the public health nurse, she may further delay screening and intervention and adversely affect her health status. Variant cultural values and fears must be acknowledged by the public health nurse as it relates to cancer diagnosis and prognosis. Particular minority groups are known to delay diagnosis and treatment until advance disease. Religious convictions also influence certain decisions about accessing healthcare services.

Too often, nurses isolate their services to the primary client and do not respond to the needs and interests of other family members. This practice limits the scope of practice and lessens the positive effects of holistic public health nursing services. Developing a comprehensive plan of care for one client should include others who are part of his or her world. These women's lives are intertwined. What happens to one influences the other. While eliciting the health and social history of Ms. L. and conducting the family assessment, the astute public health nurse will begin to incorporate the needs of other family members into a holistic plan of care (particularly Mrs. S.).

The public health nurse must expand her view of the client constellation and be attentive to the health and social needs of significant others. In addition, the need to develop a community perspective is critical. Mrs. S. has provided some clues that the PHN should investigate. She indicates a knowledge about other minority women in the immediate neighborhood with breast cancer. Questions arise. Did these women defer diagnosis and treatment until disease was advanced? Are they currently in therapy? Are there local support groups and advocates? Are there ongoing community needs?

And as such needs are identified, the public health nurse moves to the next step—incorporating the community in the plan of care. It is this common sense and comprehensive approach that allows health dividends to be experienced at the individual as well as the community level.

ANNOTATED REFERENCES

Capers, C. (1994). Mental health issues and African-Americans. *Mental Health Nursing, 29*(1), 57–64.

Issues regarding the provision of culturally appropriate and sensitive mental health nursing services to African Americans are delineated in this article. The sections on cultural awareness, cultural knowledge, cultural skill, cultural encounter, and cultural competence clarify five pertinent issues. Capers categorizes these as: personal views and historical and social factors that influence diagnosis and treatment of African Americans; influence of racism in psychiatric situations; the development of cultural understanding and skills; the recognition of intragroup commonalties and differences; and the evolution of health policies to provide culturally appropriate mental health services to diverse groups.

Healthy People 2000: National Health Objectives: Black Americans. (1991). *U.S. Department of Health and Human Services, Public Health Service,* 1–11.

This Healthy People 2000 (HP2000) report highlights national health objectives targeting Black Americans. Its objectives support the overall HP 2000 goals that are to: increase the span of healthy life for Americans, reduce health disparities among Americans, and achieve access to preventive services for all Americans. African Americans make up more than 12 percent of the United States population and constitute the nation's largest minority group. Black Americans are at particular risk for premature disability and death in comparison to the general population. This report is to be used in conjunction with the full set of Healthy People 2000 objectives and the midcourse Review released by the Secretary of Health, U.S. Department of Health and Human Services.

Mack, E., McGrath, T., Pendleton, D., & Zieber, N. (1993). Reaching poor populations with cancer prevention and early detection programs. *Cancer Practice,* *1*(1), 35–39.

This article describes the collaborative educational, professional, and organizational approach to provide cancer prevention and early detection programs to economically disadvantaged women in one urban setting. Creative interventions address the inequity in cancer education and access to working poor, culturally diverse women. Successful strategies include outreach, teaching modules, available staff for professional and public education and consultation, and onsite translators.

Moormeier, J. (1996). Breast cancer in black women. *Annuals of Internal Medicine,* *124*(10), 897–905.

Moormeir reviews current knowledge about breast cancer in African American women using MEDLINE as the data source from 1966 to 1995. This review documents the discrepancy in survival rate between African American and white women. African American women present at time of diagnosis with more advanced disease, with tumors that are different than in white women (and less receptive to therapies) and with confounding comorbid conditions and socioeconomic factors. The author emphasizes the need to improve efforts in community education, early screening efforts and early detection for African American women, particularly those who are poor, elderly, or without a consistent source of healthcare.

Morrison, C. (1996). Using PRECEDE to predict breast self-examination in older, lower-income women. *American Journal of Health Behavior, 20*(2), 3–14.

Morrison uses the PRECEDE framework to organize potential predictors of breast self-examination (BSE) in an effort to identify factors which are associated with BSE in 204 older, low-income women. Study limitations are identified. Ten influential factors supporting regular BSE are discussed. These include the woman's educational level, BSE skill mastery, confidence in self-efficacy, awareness of mammography as diagnostic tool, risk factor knowledge, taught time of month to perform BSE, and the influence of provider as educator.

Powe, B. (1996). Cancer fatalism among African-Americans: A review of the literature. *Nursing Outlook, 44*(1), 18–21.

Powe's article focuses on high risk African American populations and the barrier of cancer fatalism to participation in cancer screening. The article is organized into three sections: philosophic origins of cancer fatalism among African Americans; research findings regarding cancer fatalism; implications for nursing science. Powe suggests that education interventions may not be consistently effective and that interventions must incorporate knowledge of the person's attitudes, values, and beliefs. More research in assessing the presence of cancer fatalism across the life span is necessary.

Chapter 6

PREVENTION STRATEGIES

Patricia Gerrity

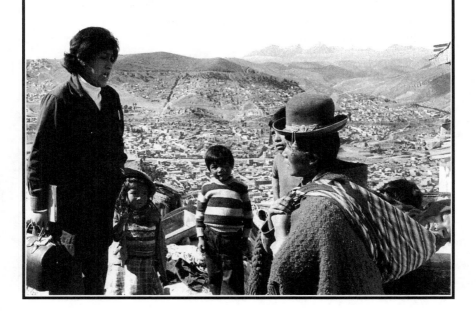

COMMENTARY

Vernice D. Ferguson

Significant challenges await the nurse as care is provided in the community. Dr. Gerrity identifies two major public health problems in the two case studies presented: preventing childhood poisoning and improving immunization rates in marginalized children. These problems become a potent reminder that a broader conceptualization of health is required. All too often health and illness care have been viewed narrowly and as a single entity.

In managed care settings and as healthcare takes on a larger community focus, health promotion and disease prevention become important functions for nurses. The impact of the environment and lifestyle on health status takes on new meaning. The nurse soon recognizes that involvement in the community is essential as new partnerships are forged with various community organizations to improve the public's health. Creative approaches and new skills are required as effective involvement of all relevant entities in a given community and beyond its borders are mobilized to address environmental concerns and prevailing lifestyles that affect a population's health status.

We can learn from successful models. Hence, more nurses must become knowledgeable about public health approaches. Continuing education for many nurses must now be broadened to include attendance at major meetings of public health organizations and reading in the field of public health.

Preventing Childhood Lead Poisoning

OBJECTIVES

---

1. Discuss ways to prevent lead exposure in young children.
2. Identify multilevel approaches to improving immunization status in a community.
3. Describe the role of community organizations in health prevention programs.
4. Examine the relationship between routine well child care and screening programs.

*D*oretha Marshall is a public health nurse working at a nurse-managed center in Walnut Hill, a large urban community. Census data indicate that the population is 73 percent African American, 10 percent Caucasian, and 17 percent immigrants, many of whom are undocumented. The rate of births to single mothers is 72 percent and 67 percent live at or below the poverty level. The few small industries that were in the area have closed, reducing the number of jobs and leaving many abandoned buildings.

There are several large hospitals in areas contiguous with Walnut Hill and a few private physicians. There is one city health center that offers primary care services, but no public health nursing services. Although 68 percent of the children are Medicaid eligible, only half have received EPSDT (early periodic screening diagnosis and treatment) services in the past year. Childhood lead poisoning continues to be a problem, along with inadequate immunization rates in preschool children. Informal surveys indicate that many private physicians are not aware of the revised guidelines from the Centers for Disease Control regarding screening for lead poisoning in children.

The director of the local Head Start Program approaches Doretha requesting that she provide lead screening for the children in her program. Health department data for the area indicates a general reduction in lead levels overall, but an increase in the number of children who demonstrate levels in the 10 to 20 microgram range. (Normally no lead is detected, levels <10mg/dl are considered normal.) In 1993, 445 of children tested had lead poisoning almost five times the national average.

Last year, Doretha attended an environmental health seminar and learned that lead poisoning is preventable with low-tech methods of lead reduction. The single most effective protective measure is to have children wash their hands frequently with regular soap. Floors and household surfaces should be washed weekly using a phosphate detergent, since vacuuming or dusting can just spread lead dust.

Doretha knows of a program in another neighborhood in the same city, that employed workers who went door to door to test for lead dust in homes, and offer screening to young children, along with educational materials. This program had difficulty reaching the intended population. Many people were reluctant to let the workers into their homes.

QUESTIONS

1. How might Doretha respond to the Head Start director's request for lead screening?
2. How is lead screening performed? What issues are involved in determining who is to be screened?
3. What is the role of the public health department in lead screening? In regard to EPSDT?
4. What are some potential explanations for people's reluctance to let the lead team into their homes?
5. How might Doretha learn more about these concerns?
6. What more might Doretha want to know about the EPSDT program?
7. What groups in the community might join forces to prevent childhood lead poisoning?
8. What groups might be threatened by these actions?

ANALYSIS AND DISCUSSION

Childhood lead poisoning is one of the most common pediatric health problems in the United States today, and it is entirely preventable. Lead poisoning, for the most part, is silent; most poisoned children have no symptoms. The vast majority of cases, therefore, go undiagnosed and untreated.

Lead poisoning is widespread, it is not solely a problem of inner city or minority children.

In the past several years, scientific evidence shows that some adverse effects occur at blood lead levels at least as low as 10 micrograms/dl in children. This evidence has become so overwhelming and compelling that it has become a major force in determining how we approach childhood lead exposure. Primary prevention efforts need to be increasingly focused on preventing lead poisoning before it occurs. This requires community-wide, environmental interventions, as well as educational and nutritional campaigns.

Eradicating childhood lead poisoning requires a long-term active program of primary lead poisoning prevention, including abatement of lead-based paint hazards in homes, daycare centers and other places where young children play and live. Prevention programs at the community level require the support and cooperation of a number of participants at various levels, from the families themselves to landlords and legislators.

The most effective action that families can take is to remove potential lead dust from the home by cleaning with phosphate soap, and by washing children's hands and toys. This eliminates much of the exposure in young children. However, many families are sensitive to the fact they live in homes which are in ill repair and have little resources with which to make necessary changes. The nurse must be particularly sensitive to the fact that in trying to teach families specific ways of cleaning their homes, they are not making assumptions about the house cleaning abilities of the parents. In addition, many families are in tenuous situations regarding their housing and are afraid that their landlords, or family members from which they rent space, will insist that they move out rather than face the cost of lead abatement. The nurse must work closely with groups and agencies in the community with whom she can gain support for communitywide prevention approaches.

The public health nurse has a major role to play in both preventing and screening for lead poisoning in children. Screening should be a routine part of well child care for children ages 1 to 6 years. Children who are not routinely screened may also not be receiving other important components of EPSDT programs or not be in the program at all. It would be helpful for the nurse to speak with the director of the Head Start program about helping to link families to routine, continuous sources of primary care rather than do testing for lead and other required problems separate from the children's routine care.

ANNOTATED REFERENCES

Centers for Disease Control. (1991). *Preventing lead poisoning in young children* (A statement by the Centers for Disease Control). Atlanta: Author.

This comprehensive review of childhood lead poisoning can be used as a basic reference for information about lead poisoning in general, screening, sources and pathways of lead exposure, the role of providers and agencies, as well as management of lead toxicity at both the individual and community levels. The recommendations are based mainly on the scientific data showing adverse effects of lead in young children at increasingly lower blood lead levels. They are tempered, however, by practical considerations, for example, of the numbers of children who would require follow-up and the resources required to prevent the disease.

Simons-Morton, D. G., Simons-Morton, B. G., & Parcel, G. S. (1988). Influencing personal and environmental conditions for community health: A multi-level intervention model. *Family Community Health, 11*(2), 25–35.

The importance of both personal and environmental conditions to health are discussed. The authors then present a multilevel intervention model for practical use in influencing both conditions. Applications of the model are presented to illustrate how the model can be used. The model has proven particularly valuable in sorting out the target population from the targets of intervention and in conceptualizing the range of possible intervention approaches.

Improving Immunization Rates

1. Identify the major indicators of children's health status.
2. Discuss the role of the health department in disease prevention.
3. Identify the cultural aspects of care for diverse populations.

A local civic group recently approached a nurse-managed health center in a large urban area about the possibility of providing funds to support a one-day immunization drive. The staff at the center have been concerned about the immunization status of this population, particularly in the Southeast Asian children, and would like financial support for their current and future efforts. But from their previous experience with immunization campaigns they know that a great deal of work goes into preparing a one-day event, and the turnout in this community has been poor.

The nurse does not want to turn down the offer of financial support for this important health problem, but she knows that more sustained efforts are needed to be effective in addressing the problem.

The targeted neighborhood has declined in total population over the past ten years. The housing is mostly renter occupied, with many abandoned homes, and illegal occupancy. There is only one remaining factory in the area in which the work is seasonal and leaving many workers periodically without benefits such as health insurance.

There is one teaching hospital on the periphery of the neighborhood, but it is not seen as welcoming by the local residents. The hospital has made efforts to collaborate with the community organizations, but its long history of paternalism and lack of cultural sensitivity to the changing population has blocked these efforts.

The population consists of African American, Caribbean, Korean, Hmong, Cambodian, Vietnamese, and Laotian families. The local elementary school has identified 22 languages spoken among the families. There is one Asian physician with an office in the community and many ethnic and civic associations. There is an active network of block associations, mostly composed of African Americans, many of whom have a long history of activism in this community.

QUESTIONS

1. What additional information does the nurse need about this community?
2. What are the possible sources for the information?
3. How would the nurse begin to form a coalition to address the problem?
4. What agencies/community groups might get involved and why?
5. Comment on the position of the local hospital.
6. How might the nurse approach the civic group who offers assistance?
7. What is known about immunization status? How would the nurse find out?
8. What is the role of the health department?

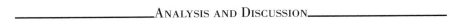

ANALYSIS AND DISCUSSION

Reaching minority families to link them with a medical home and improve their immunization rates continues to be one of the most challenging issues facing communities. Minority families are disproportionately affected by underimmunization, mainly by virtue of their lower socioeconomic status and limited access to health services. Compounding these factors are a variety of cultural differences that influence minority families' health choices.

Much has been documented about income and its relationship to poor health status. Families living at or below the poverty level are less likely to have health insurance, less educated, younger, and more likely to be single-parent, usually mother-only. However, while vaccination levels are worst among low-income, urban, non-White children, all groups of children are behind in getting their shots. Minority families, especially recent immigrants, often have difficulty accessing health services, due to the location and hours of health clinics. Keeping track of complicated immunization schedules is also a challenge. Compounding the problem is a lack of adequate health information and educational materials written in different languages that are simple to follow, yet retain respect for the parents' intelligence.

The nurse must conduct a thorough assessment of the target population and the environment in which they live to create a successful outreach strategy. Community representatives should be consulted to determine the particular concerns and be engaged from the outset in designing strategies for improving awareness. It is wise to draw people from the target communities to be part of an outreach team. People who are of the same cultural, racial, and ethnic background will be better able to communicate the importance of immunization and other primary care issues and help build trust and confidence in the healthcare system. In many cultures, the support and respect of community leaders must be won in order to open effective channels of communication.

Culturally appropriate messages and materials must take into account the language generally spoken and the community's beliefs and attitudes regarding immunization, healthcare, and the providers in the area.

It is important for the nurse to know that one-time or one-day campaigns are not effective in improving immunization rates. Programs need to be ongoing and link children to a routine source of primary care. The nurse may have to educate the local civic group about the effectiveness of "campaigns" and help them to channel their funding into more productive and cost effective strategies.

ANNOTATED REFERENCES

Freed, G., Bordley, W., & Defriese, G. (1993). Childhood immunization programs: An analysis of policy issues. *Milbank Quarterly, 71*(1), 65–96.

Examines the current state of childhood immunization in this country and offers a broad range of suggestions for policy modification. It begins with a background of vaccine rates for children comparing the rates in the United States to those in other countries. It then goes into detailed descriptions of the four problems and their solutions: (1) access problems for patients; (2) barriers in both public and private sectors; (3) compliance with existing vaccine recommendations; and (4) development of new vaccines.

Immunizing America's children: Strategies and partnerships to remove the barriers to immunization. (1995). Children's Action Network.

A compilation of strategies and approaches that have led to real success in communities across the country. It provides a comprehensive framework for organizations and coalitions that want to remove the barriers to immunization. It also summarizes the practical steps that a variety of different organizations in diverse communities across the country have found effective.

Chapter 7

PROVIDING RELEVANT CARE:
Values and Valuing

Donna Faust Patterson

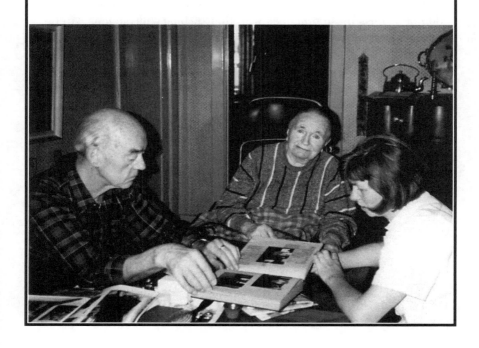

COMMENTARY

Vernice D. Ferguson

As healthcare costs are rationalized, we can expect to see more home care emerge, especially as chronic conditions are managed at home and with greater involvement of the family. The challenge for nurses is to develop mastery in comprehensive discharge planning. Early discharges from hospitals are the norm and Maria's case demonstrates the new reality. Faculty members play a major role as they assist students in determining what requires attention and when, for both the students and family care givers can become overwhelmed with all that presents itself in the home environment.

Dr. Patterson assists us in appreciating the importance of making a culturally relevant assessment based on knowledge of a cultural group's shared values and beliefs. In all three case studies, she reminds us that when working with culturally diverse groups their prevailing health practices must be respected as trust is built.

We have come to realize that increasingly more westerners are using alternative or complementary therapies. In the United States, it has been estimated that one out of three individuals uses some form of alternative therapy, while seven in ten users of alternative therapy do not discuss these practices with their primary physicians. An office for alternative medicine now exists at the National Institutes of Health. Funded programs are in place and major conferences held related to alternative healthcare practices. At some of the conferences, demonstrations and practicums are offered. Curricula in some health professional schools reflect this new occurrence in course work.

Eisenberg, D. M., Kessler, R. C., Foster, C., Norlock, F. E., Calkins, D. R., & Delbanco, T. L. (1993). Unconventional medicine in the United States—prevalence, costs and patterns of use: Results of a national survey. *New England Journal of Medicine, 328:*246–252.

Developmental Disability Requiring Home Care

OBJECTIVES
---

1. To identify the assessment data required prior to Maria's discharge to develop a comprehensive family nursing care plan.
2. To plan effective nursing interventions for Maria and her family once she has returned home.
3. To address the unique needs of the family by incorporating culturally relevant assessment and nursing care into discharge and home care planning.

*M*aria A. is a 9-month-old female who was born at 29 weeks gestation and suffered anoxia at birth. She is the third child of Jose and Carmen. Their other two children are Anamaria who is 6-years-old and Jesus who is 4-years-old. They live in a three-bedroom apartment on the third floor of an apartment building in New York City. Carmen's mother, Estella, lives on the second floor with one teenage son and her own mother. The family speaks Spanish at home. They attend mass regularly at the local Roman Catholic church. The family was often accompanied on hospital visits by a family friend who practiced the healing art, *curanderismo*.

Maria's first hospitalization lasted four months. She was discharged from the intensive care nursery to home where her family cared for her until she suffered aspiration pneumonia one month ago. She is now being prepared for discharge to home from the pediatric unit. Maria is unable to roll over or sit, she makes no sounds, and her pupils respond slowly to light. She does not suck, has no grasp reflex, and withdraws from pain. She has a tracheostomy and has difficulty handling secretions requiring frequent suctioning. She has been diagnosed with severe developmental delay, tonic-clonic and partial seizures, gastroesophageal reflux with esophagitis, and has a gastrostomy tube for feeding. Maria's family is anxiously awaiting her return. The hospitalization has disrupted their family routine.

The nurse has determined that the family immigrated from Mexico 10 years ago. Jose is employed as a taxi cab driver in the evenings. Carmen works in a fast-food restaurant as a cook during the breakfast shift. Estella works in the local grocery store as a clerk. Anamaria and Jesus attend the school program at the parish church.

Her orders include:

1. Bolus feedings 150cc of formula four times per day followed by 100 cc of water.
2. Postural drainage and percussion every four hours.
3. Suctioning as needed.
4. Medications:
   Ranitidine syrup 85 mg, GT BID
   Carbamazepine oral suspension, 200 mg, GT, TID
   Ferrous Sulfate oral solution 30 mg, GT BID

Consider the following questions in preparing Maria for discharge and the early home visits by the home health nurse.

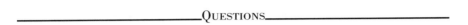

QUESTIONS

1. Describe the religious and cultural practices that might influence Maria's care.
2. What are potential etiologies of Maria's disorders?
3. What priority nursing assessments need to be completed at the first home visit considering Maria's diagnosis and the specialized medical devices she requires?
4. Explain the care a tracheostomy tube and gastrostomy tube require.
5. What are the purposes and side effects of each medication?
6. Considering their ages and stages of development, describe the effects of Maria's chronic illness on her siblings, Anamaria and Jesus.
7. What are Carmen and Jose's anticipated needs for home care, assessment of potential illnesses or problems, maintenance of their own emotional well-being, and providing a nurturing environment for their children?
8. What services are available in your community for developmentally delayed children and their families?

ANALYSIS AND DISCUSSION

This analysis focuses on consideration of barriers to health care faced by people of diverse cultures and the complexity of care required by technologically dependent children. Kohn (1995) identifies four barriers to culturally competent care:

1. American medicine is an alien culture.
2. Native language is not spoken by healthcare providers.
3. Customs are not understood or respected.
4. Trust is difficult to establish given the current healthcare system.

Technologically dependent children require highly skilled physical care within the context of their family unit and their culture.

Maria is returning to her home. Her family will assume responsibility for her physical and emotional care within the context of their value, religious, and cultural systems. The Anglo-American healthcare system may only partially meet the family's needs by diagnosing and treating the physical problems (airway obstruction leading to tracheostomy, esophageal reflux and altered feeding patterns, seizures, and developmental delay). It is helpful for the nurses involved in care to recognize the religious belief system and the meaning of bearing and caring for a chronically ill child in the Mexican American culture. Mexican Americans may view chronic illness as God's punishment for past transgressions, illness as a manifestation of strong emotion, or being out of balance. Given these alternative views of illness causation, the family's methods for managing illness states may differ from the Anglo health-care system's recommendation (Clark, 1996; Elfert, Anderson, & Lai, 1991).

Both spoken word and nonverbal communication may thwart communication between people of different ethnic backgrounds. Native language can be accommodated through bilingual staff members or trained interpreters. Family members may prefer to bring their own interpreter. Parents may not be the only family members involved in the decision-making process about Maria's care. Cultures with different hierarchial relationships may bestow the greatest influence on the grandparent, father, or elder in the community. Mothers may be consulted at the bedside, but need to consult others before making decisions about their child's care. Effective nurses are sensitive to cues from children and families that the message presented is supportive and helpful (Jackson, 1993).

Maria's family practices *curanderismo,* a healing art based on the belief that God heals through people who have been given the special gift of healing. Nurses who recognize and support families who practice healing rituals unfamiliar to Anglo healthcare providers have the opportunity to develop a more open and trusting relationship. Nurses can support cultural practices by providing privacy, allowing the intervention to occur, and providing time for families to discuss their feelings and practices if they so choose. Interventions directed toward meeting the unique needs of families will aid in developing a trusting relationship.

_____ANNOTATED REFERENCES_____

Clark, M. (1995, May/June). Biomedicine, meet ethnomedicine. *Healthcare Forum Journal,* 20–29.

The author discusses the need for culturally sensitive healthcare. She provides an overview of culturally specific concepts of health such as *curanderismo* (Mexican), *nizone* (Navajo), and *qi* (Chinese), reviews several community programs that have been successful in integrating culturally sensitive care, and lists examples of open-ended questions that health providers might ask to better understand the meaning of the illness to the patient.

Clark, M. J. (1996). Cultural influences on community health. In *Nursing in the Community* (2nd ed., pp. 273–340). Stamford, CT: Appleton & Lange.

This textbook chapter supplies an overview of health and dietary practices of several prevalent American subcultures. The information is useful and readily applicable to clinical situations.

Elfert, H., Anderson, J. M., & Lai, M. (1991). Parent's perceptions of children with chronic illness: A study of immigrant Chinese families. *Journal of Pediatric Nursing, 6*(2), 114–120.

This phenomenological research describes the differences in interpretation of chronic illness between Euro-Canadian families and Chinese immigrant families. The Chinese families attribute more global effects of illness to the child and future possibilities. The research demonstrates the need to understand the subculture's interpretation of illness in planning future care.

Jackson, L. E. (1993). Understanding, eliciting, and negotiating client's multicultural beliefs. *Nurse Practitioner, 18*(4), 30–43.

The author describes the interconnectedness of cultural beliefs and healing. She explains the clinical encounter and how nurses can elicit culturally specific information using open-ended questions. Finally, she gives examples of several case studies and how they were influenced by the individual's culture.

Kohn, S. (1995, May/June). Dismantling sociocultural barriers to care. *Healthcare Forum Journal,* 30–33.

This article describes four sociocultural barriers to healthcare: (1) American medicine as alien culture, (2) language barriers, (3) customs and beliefs are not understood or respected, and (4) lack of mutual trust. The article goes on to list strategies that may be helpful to minimize barriers such as partnering with the community and making the clinic a welcoming place.

Dealing with Upper Respiratory Infections

—————————————OBJECTIVES—————————————

1. To identify culturally specific practices in various healthcare settings.
2. To value cultural differences acting in ways to maintain individual and family integrity.
3. To evaluate culturally specific practices in view of the overriding American culture.

*L*oan is a 6-month-old Vietnamese girl who was brought to the clinic by her mother because she has a runny nose and has been hot for three days. Her mother is accompanied by a friend who speaks English. Loan was born in the United States (her mother and father were born in Vietnam). Her mother had the usual prenatal care and an uncomplicated birth. The baby has completed her 2-month and 4-month immunizations at the clinic. Loan lives with her father, mother, paternal grandparents, two sisters (4 years and 3 years of age), and a great uncle. The family runs a small community grocery store.

Loan's temperature is 38.9°C, her nasal drainage is yellow and thick. She is irritable and shaking her head back and forth. She has been refusing rice soup, formula, and sweet tea.

During the intake interview, the nurse notices small red bruises on the baby's temples and center of the forehead above the nose. The nurse notes the mother has small bandage-type plasters applied to her temples. The baby smells faintly of lemon.

The mother is talking quietly to her daughter, rocking her, and trying to offer her tea with sugar from a bottle. The friend who acts as the interpreter is consulting with the mother and responding to the nurse's questions in English. The interpreter tells the nurse that Loan's grandmother wanted to call in a healer who practiced cupping to cure the baby. Loan's mother was afraid it would hurt her.

Bilateral otitis media is found on physical examination. Amoxicillin 125 mg per 5 ml is prescribed three times per day for 10 days.

Consider the following questions while developing a nursing care plan for Loan and her family.

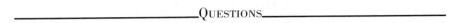

QUESTIONS

1. What health practices specific to the Vietnamese culture are identified by the clinic nurse?
2. List associated health practices not mentioned that may cause unusual skin symptoms.
3. What is the usual family structure in this culture? Who would health-care workers address to enlist help to implement a healthcare plan?
4. Discuss health practices and home remedies in your own subculture that may impact on acceptance of healthcare prescriptions.
5. Review family structure and hierarchical structure in your own subculture that may impact on the delivery of healthcare.

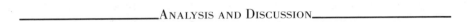

ANALYSIS AND DISCUSSION

This analysis focuses on consideration of barriers to healthcare faced by people of diverse cultures and the need to recognize folk-healing practices as legitimate self-care activities in caring for a sick child. Kohn (1995) identifies four barriers to culturally competent care: (1) American medicine is an alien culture; (2) native language is not spoken by healthcare providers; 3) customs are not understood or respected; and (4) trust is difficult to establish given the current healthcare system.

The family structure is based on paternal lineage. The oldest living male is the head of household. When that man dies, his eldest son assumes family responsibility. Traditionally, women take residence with and the name of their husband's family. They assume household responsibilities as directed by their mother-in-law. Child care is the women's domain; consultation about daily matters occurs among the women. Respect for elders is key. Young people are expected to turn to their elders to make decisions. Therefore, decisions about children's healthcare may be mandated by the grandmother or grandfather. Decisions such as hospitalization are often deferred to the head of household.

Some generalizations can be made about the Vietnamese culture's concept of health. Most Asian American beliefs about maintaining health are related to ancient Chinese medicine where care is focused on achieving balance of the life force. Disease is caused by soul loss, spiritual possession, breach of taboo, object intrusion, or an imbalance of *Yin* and *Yang* (*Am* and *Duong* in Vietnamese). Diseases are classified as hot or cold. Treatments are complimentary. Characteristics of foods are ascribed to hot and cold and foods are chosen or avoided during times of illness depending on the disease. Blood is considered irreplaceable and, if lost, part of the spirit is lost. Consequently, the family may resist blood drawing for tests. The Asian cultures respect Western medical practice; however, they may not report seeking help from a healer within their own culture out of respect for both practitioners (Clark, 1996). Many of these concepts do not translate easily to English and it may be difficult to help the Western healthcare practitioner understand the Asian family's beliefs and customs. It may also be difficult to provide an anatomy based explanation of the illness because Asian cultures do not view body function from a Western, scientific standpoint.

It is estimated that 70 percent of treatments for illness are initiated and carried out by the individual or a significant other without consulting a health professional. These practices vary among groups and depend on things such as knowledge level, belief system, and cultural background. In this instance, Loan's mother with the help of family members attempted to treat her fever using several traditional Vietnamese remedies. The Vietnamese culture uses several techniques to treat symptoms prior to seeking the advice of western healthcare professionals. They include acupuncture, herbal medicines and teas, balancing hot and cold foods, acupressure, massage, meditation, cupping, pinching. steaming, coining, and moxibustion (Clark, 1996). This family attempted to alleviate the fever with cold foods, herbal teas, mentholated plasters, pinching, and massage with lemon. Western medicine is considered potent, requiring only small doses of medication to relieve symptoms. This family may need specific instructions about the dose and use antibiotics so that Loan is treated adequately. The probability of successful treatment will be enhanced by understanding and respecting cultural differences, supporting traditional care giver activities that are not unsafe, and resisting imposition of the western view of health exclusive of traditional healthcare practices.

ANNOTATED REFERENCES

Andrews, M. M., & Boyle, J. S. (1995). *Transcultural concepts in nursing care* (2nd ed.). Philadelphia: Lippincott.
This book provides a clear explanation of transcultural nursing care. The chapters include information on theoretical underpinnings, developmental needs, family

differences, and community and religious influences of culture on individuals. It also gives direction to culturally appropriate nursing care.

Clark, M. (1995, May/June). Biomedicine, meet ethnomedicine. *Healthcare Forum Journal*, 20–29.

The author discusses the need for culturally sensitive health care. She provides an overview of culturally specific concepts of health such as *curanderismo* (Mexican), *nizone* (Navajo), and *qi* (Chinese), reviews several community programs that have been successful in integrating culturally sensitive care, and lists examples of open-ended questions that health providers might ask to better understand the meaning of the illness to the patient.

Clark, M. J. (1996). Cultural influences on community health. In *Nursing in the community* (2nd ed., pp. 273–340). Stamford, CT: Appleton & Lange.

This textbook chapter supplies an overview of health and dietary practices of several prevalent American subcultures. The information is useful and readily applicable to clinical situations.

Elfert, H., Anderson, J. M., & Lai, M. (1991). Parent's perceptions of children with chronic illness: A study of immigrant Chinese families. *Journal of Pediatric Nursing, 6*(2), 114–120.

This phenomenological research describes the differences in interpretation of chronic illness between Euro-Canadian families and Chinese immigrant families. The Chinese families attribute more global effects of illness to the child and future possibilities. The research demonstrates the need to understand the subculture's interpretation of illness in planning future care.

Jackson, L. E. (1993). Understanding, eliciting, and negotiating client's multicultural beliefs. *Nurse Practitioner, 18*(4), 30–43.

The author describes the interconnectedness of cultural beliefs and healing. She explains the clinical encounter and how nurses can elicit culturally specific information using open-ended questions. Finally, she gives examples of several case studies and how they were influenced by the individual's culture.

Kohn, S. (1995, May/June). Dismantling sociocultural barriers to care. *Healthcare Forum Journal*, 30–33.

This article describes four sociocultural barriers to healthcare: (1) American medicine as alien culture, (2) language barrier, (3) customs and beliefs are not understood or respected, and (4) lack of mutual trust. The article lists strategies that may be helpful to minimize barriers such as partnering with the community and making the clinic a welcoming place.

School Nurse in an Inner City School

1. To review health promotion goals.
2. To plan age and culturally appropriate health education materials for school-age children.

*T*he school nurse is assigned to a new school in her district. It is an elementary school (kindergarten through 5th grade) whose students and families are ethnically diverse. The median family income is $15,000, many children live in single parent households or with grandparents or other relatives. More than 35 percent of the students are considered overweight. Physical education classes are held only once a week for each grade and many students are afraid to play outdoors after school. Drug activity and gang violence have been reported in the neighborhood; however, a neighborhood watch program is being organized. About one-third of the students classify themselves as African American, one third as Hispanic, and one third as Asian heritage. About half the students qualify for the school meal program.

It is the nurse's task to plan a comprehensive health promotion program that can be presented to students in each class on a weekly basis. The goals of the health promotion program are to be based on Healthy People 2000 (USPHS, 1990). The program is to encourage practice of healthy behaviors with age-appropriate activities and to improve students' knowledge of healthy behaviors.

The local university's nursing department has adopted this school and will be assisting the school nurse in planning and implementing the health promotion program.

1. Identify four healthy behaviors that are appropriate to each grade level (be cognizant of developmental expectations and at-risk behaviors for each age group).

2. Choose one healthy behavior for each grade level and design a 20-minute activity to teach that concept. Include a lesson plan, materials list, and outcomes for the activity.
3. List food staples and preferences for each of the cultural groups. Identify the heart healthy components of each diet.
4. Plan a heart healthy meal for each cultural group listed. Identify a grade level and describe how you might incorporate this meal plan into a classroom activity.
5. Plan one activity for a parent group to improve parenting skills, provide information about developmental changes in children, or encourage incorporation of a healthy lifestyle change into a family's routine.

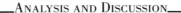

ANALYSIS AND DISCUSSION

This analysis focuses on consideration of barriers to health faced by people of diverse cultures and the identified national goals for health promotion (USPHS, 1990). Kohn (1995) identifies four barriers to culturally competent care: (1) American medicine is an alien culture, (2) native language is not spoken by healthcare providers, (3) customs are not understood or respected, and (4) trust is difficult to establish given the current healthcare system.

In this case study, the community is the client and the community has multiple health-related needs. Examples of health promotion needs include exercise and fitness, nutrition, avoidance of substance abuse, family planning, and violence prevention. Each of these health promotion goals could be a year-long focus activity for the school or for specific grade levels. Lessons could then be designed to build knowledge and skills in these areas. It is necessary to plan activities that are age and grade appropriate, involve all the students, and allow for their input. The diversity of cultural backgrounds will expand the challenge to address the broad-based needs of the community. Each cultural group views health differently, practices health behaviors according to their traditions, and defines health prevention behaviors according to their unique experience.

To integrate the culturally diverse groups and address varying needs, it is important to plan activities to include all children and parents who will be involved. One specific area where these groups differ substantially is food choice and preparation. To understand the nutritional needs of these children, one must first understand their dietary practices, determine strengths and areas of concern in dietary intake of each culture, and then help to choose the healthy foods for that culture.

Nutritional habits established in childhood are being implicated in cardiovascular disease, cancer, and hypertension. It is especially important to recognize the influence of these early eating habits on obesity, hypertension, and heart disease in adulthood.

Food not only nourishes the body, but is often the center of family gatherings and celebrations. Foods return us to our family of origin and maintains connections. Spices such as ginger and garlic are associated with Asian cuisine and cilantro with Mexican fare. In view of these cultural connections, it is necessary for nurses and nutritionists to consider how to establish healthy eating habits within the culture's food preferences.

ANNOTATED REFERENCES

Andrews, M. M., & Boyle, J. S. (1995). *Transcultural concepts in nursing care* (2nd ed.). Philadelphia: Lippincott.

This book provides a clear explanation of transcultural nursing care. The chapters include information on theoretical underpinnings, developmental needs, family differences, and community and religious influences of culture on individuals. It also gives direction to culturally appropriate nursing care.

Clark, M. J. (1996). Cultural influences on community health. In *Nursing in the community* (2nd ed., pp. 273–340). Stamford, CT: Appleton & Lange.

This textbook chapter supplies an overview of health and dietary practices of several prevalent American subcultures. The information is useful and readily applicable to clinical situations.

Jackson, L. E. (1993). Understanding, eliciting, and negotiating client's multicultural beliefs. *Nurse Practitioner, 18*(4), 30–43.

The author describes the interconnectedness of cultural beliefs and healing. She explains the clinical encounter and how nurses can elicit culturally specific information using open ended questions. Finally, she gives examples of several case studies and how they were influenced by the individual's culture.

Kohn, S. (1995, May/June). Dismantling sociocultural barriers to care. *Healthcare Forum Journal,* 30–33.

This article describes four sociocultural barriers to healthcare: (1) American medicine as alien culture, (2) language barrier, (3) customs and beliefs are not understood or respected, and (4) lack of mutual trust. The article lists strategies that may be helpful to minimize barriers such as partnering with the community and making the clinic a welcoming place.

U.S. Public Health Service. (1990). *Healthy people 2000: National health promotion and disease prevention objectives* (Doc. # PHS 91-50213). Washington, DC: U.S. Government Printing Office.

This document sets out a framework to prevent major chronic diseases, injuries, and infectious diseases in the United States. The health promotion objectives address physical activity, nutrition, tobacco, alcohol and drugs, family planning, mental health, violence, and community-based health programs.

Chapter 8

THE CHALLENGE OF HOME CARE

Donna Tartasky

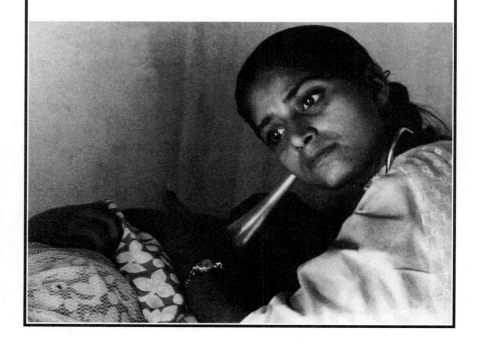

COMMENTARY

Vernice D. Ferguson

Home care is a rapidly growing and largely unregulated part of the healthcare delivery system. The process of assessment of care needs in the home is of utmost importance. Unlike the hospital where several providers have contact with a patient in a day, the home is unique in that only one nurse may see a patient in a given day. If something is omitted or a significant finding goes unnoticed, there is no other nurse who is available as in a hospital setting to assess the patient's needs. In these case studies, Dr. Tartasky underscores the importance of performing a comprehensive assessment as two patients are admitted for home care services. The pivotal role of the nurse in discharge planning and the management of care is stressed.

Assessing the Home Care Patient

_____OBJECTIVES_____

1. Understand the role of the care manager or discharge planner in coordinating service delivery.
2. Identify interdisciplinary services that would assist the client and family.
3. Describe the process of assessment in a home care setting.

*T*he process of assessment in the home is of utmost importance. Unlike the hospital where several providers have contact with any one patient in a day, the home is unique in that only one nurse may see a patient in a given day. If you omit something or don't notice a significant finding, remember that no one will come in on the next shift to assess the patient. The importance of this is underscored by two case studies of two patients admitted for home care services.

J.F. was a 78-year-old male admitted to home care services for skilled nursing and physical therapy evaluations. J.F. had been hospitalized for over two months, following his third cardiac bypass procedure in the past few years. Prior to this surgery, J.F. had a myocardial infarction and was forced to undergo this third bypass. Post-operatively, J.F. developed congestive heart failure and arrhythmias and he was transferred back into the intensive care unit from the rehabilitation facility. He stayed there a short time, went back through the step down unit and back again to the rehabilitation facility. Unfortunately, he repeated this process once more until he was eventually discharged home in care of his daughter, L.F., with whom he lived. Although the daughter understood what was required in her father's care, L.F. was overwhelmed by the change in her father, as he had previously been more independent. He was weak and more dependent, which necessitated her administering all his medications. Type of medications and dosages were reviewed with L.F., and a schedule was drawn up for her to administer medications. She was particularly concerned about a medication that necessitated her waking her father every six hours. Since it was a Saturday and she knew her father's internist was away until Monday, she agreed to try this schedule until then, at which time she could call the physician. Overall, J.F. was in fairly good shape. He was lucid, alert, and had stable vital signs. However, he was thin, slightly pale and somewhat cachectic due to his long hospitalization. Even though there were no significant findings identified, given his history, the nurse was uneasy about waiting until Monday for his next nursing visit. L.F. was given directions to call if necessary for a Sunday visit. After discussion with the home health supervisor it was decided that a visit would be made on Sunday. L.F. was called and told the nurse would be there the next day between 8:30 and 9:00 A.M.

The next day the door was half open when the nurse arrived, as if the occupants were anxiously awaiting the visit. J.F.'s daughter called down from upstairs telling the nurse her father was having a bad day. J.F. said he had awakened with chest pain and was unable to negotiate the steps to go downstairs that morning. He described his chest pain as midsternal pressure. He was pale, with stable vital signs. Given his history and symptoms, he needed to be sent to the emergency room for an evaluation. He had an old bottle of "leftover" nitroglycerin in the home, but hadn't used it in quite awhile. The covering physician was somewhat acquainted with J.F. and proceeded to tell the nurse over the phone that the patient had been abruptly discharged on Friday without medical clearance from his private physician. The doctor agreed that J.F. needed to be evaluated in the emergency room. J.F. was told about the need for the evaluation and he reluctantly agreed to go to the emergency room. Since J.F. was not an acute emergency, 911 services were not used. With the nurse and L.F. on each side of J.F., he was transported downstairs and into the car. L.F. was told to take J.F.'s medications along with them to the emergency room. A call later that day to L.F. revealed that J.F. was in the intensive care unit being transfused. As it turned out he was quite anemic, a fact that was noted on his hospital record and not conveyed on his home care referral.

―――――――――――――――QUESTIONS―――――――――――――――

1. What are some of the essential questions that must be answered when the home becomes the care setting? Where should the dialogue begin? Who should become involved?
2. What are some of the strategies that the homecare nurse can use to empower the family caregiver?

―――――――――――――――ANALYSIS AND DISCUSSION―――――――――――――――

This particular case study is brief but it demonstrates some of the complex health problems presented in today's healthcare environment. Unfortunately, more and more patients are discharged without communicating important information about their needs. Hospitals need to utilize care managers or discharge planners who carefully review patient records and act as their advocate. In an era of healthcare cost rationing, the need for a healthcare professional who can assess the patient's needs before discharge can have cost-saving consequences. If J.F.'s chart had been reviewed by a care manager or discharge planner, he would not have been inappropriately discharged. The costs associated with an emergency room visit and subsequent stay in the intensive care unit could have been avoided. The care manager/discharge planner works with an interdisciplinary team to coordinate service delivery (Case Management, 1995).

In this case, planning by a healthcare professional also could have prevented immediate rehospitalization. Aside from the monetary costs, rehospitalization of the chronically ill is psychologically traumatic. In addition, interdisciplinary coordination of services would have included homemaker assistance, physical therapy, and communication with the home health nurse prior to hospital discharge. The lack of care management/discharge planning here underscores the need for comprehensive assessment by the home health nurse. The role of the home health nurse is an important one, with ever increasing responsibilities. In this case, the home health nurse also needed to provide support to J.F.'s daughter who was unmarried, and his primary caretaker. As a traditional Irish American Catholic middle-aged women, she did not know how to act as an advocate for her father (Martin, 1995). The home health nurse helped support the daughter and enlist her help in taking her father back to the hospital. Similarly, part of the role of the care manager/discharge planner would have been to empower L.F. prior to her father's discharge to act as an advocate in negotiating care for her father.

_____ANNOTATED REFERENCES_____

Martin, C. (1995). Irish Americans. In Giger & Davidhizar (Eds.), *Transcultural assessment and intervention* (pp. 347–364). St. Louis: Mosby.

This chapter provides an overview of cultural factors that affect the health behaviors of Irish Americans. Recognition of differences between members of this cultural group is noted along with implications for nursing care.

Case Management Society of America. (1995). *Standards of practice for case management.* Little Rock, AR: Author.

Managing Pain

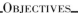
_____OBJECTIVES_____

1. Understand the role of pain management in the home.
2. Identify factors related to family caregiver stress.

*A*nother patient who was recently admitted to home care services was a 65-year-old man, J.O. The patient's wife, G.O., was downstairs and J.O. upstairs crying out for some pain medication when a nurse arrived. As G.O. explained, her husband was having pain and she had just given him some pain medication. The nurse sat with her for a few minutes, obtained written consent for the visit, and went upstairs to introduce herself to J.O. The nurse explained to J.O. that she was getting information about him from his wife and that she would spend some time with him in a little while after going over his medications with his wife. Since he had just been medicated, it was suggested he rest for awhile. The nurse checked his vital signs which were stable, positioned his head with several pillows, covered him with a blanket and went back downstairs. G.O. was tense, teary, and explained how difficult it was to manage. She told the nurse her husband had chronic renal failure and had recently been hospitalized for urinary retention and that he had also recently fractured a vertebrae. J.O. was taking about 15 medications and it took close to 1 hour with his wife to review medication dosages, names, and schedules. The nurse and G.O. then discussed how illness creates tension and she was given the opportunity to talk about her difficulties in coping. Once G.O. had the medication schedule straight, she relaxed and invited the nurse to share some holiday cookies. The nurse and G.O. spent a long time talking and then went upstairs.

Unfortunately, J.O. had to be awakened. He was quite pleasant and calmer, yet still complained of back and joint pain. The nurse explained how stress and tension are contagious between J.O. and G.O. and how they are a team and affected by each other. Much to the nurse's surprise, G.O. suddenly said that her husband had Lupus for many years. Despite having an intake record and talking with her for an hour, there had been no mention of this. Now, the pieces fit together. The nurse realized the interconnectedness of all of J.O.'s symptoms including a large inflammation of the exterior malleolus on his right ankle, that she had noticed on examination. For this patient, the need for adequate pain management was primary. If the pain was controlled, J.O. would be less tense and consequently G.O. would function better. The nurse also knew that this could not be accomplished in one visit.

Before she left, the nurse focused on what could be done immediately. Since J.O. was a big man, G.O. could not assist him in getting in and out of bed. Although he was to have a physical therapy evaluation, this would take awhile and the nurse suggested to J.O. how he could roll himself closer to the edge of the bed before getting up. Since his wife had placed a chair there, he showed the nurse how he used it to get himself to a dangling position. Fall prevention and safety were emphasized by the nurse (Lange, 1996). A schedule for pain medication was also discussed which J.O. said he would try. Once J.O. was sitting up in bed, he asked G.O. to get him a snack. The nurse accepted the offer of a beverage and spoke with J.O. while he ate. Sitting with him during his snack helped him relax, and within a short time he was quite mellow and his pain had subsided. After a total of two hours, the nurse left the house, but not before writing an extensive memo for the primary nurse about J.O., emphasizing his need for pain management and psychological support.

QUESTIONS

1. How would you develop a plan of pain management for J.O.?
2. What are the essential considerations when devising the plan?
3. What are some of the ways that the nurse can be supportive to the patient's wife? In the short-term? Over time?
4. What patient outcome should be monitored?

ANALYSIS AND DISCUSSION

One of the more interesting findings in this initial assessment and interview was the fact that J.O. had a diagnosis of Lupus that was not documented on his record or mentioned by his wife despite an indepth interview about her husband's medical history. When the diagnosis of Lupus was mentioned, the nurse realized the chronic nature of J.O.'s pain and tension. In addition to the physical assessment and interview, providing J.O. with reassurance and support were integral parts of this initial home visit. Again, in this case, the home health nurse assessed the subjective information given on the patient referral and combined that with objective data. As with the prior patient, the nurse was lacking important diagnostic information.

Caring for patient needs in the home, not unlike the hospital, is complex and requires a thorough integration of assessment, observation, and psychosocial support, as well as effective listening skills. In addition, the home health nurse needs to be prepared to alter the visit according to the patient's needs. In this case, realizing the patient had just received pain medication before she arrived, the nurse decided to take initial vital signs on J.O. and allow the medication to take effect. A comprehensive assessment was deferred for an hour, during which time the nurse collected data from G.O. and assisted in relieving her anxiety.

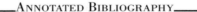

————————————ANNOTATED BIBLIOGRAPHY————————————

Lange, M. (1996). The challenge of fall prevention in home care: A review of the literature. *Home Healthcare Nurse, 14*(3), 198–206.

Falls are a leading cause of morbidity and mortality in the elderly. Identification of risk factors are discussed in this article as well as primary, secondary, and tertiary strategies that can be used by home care nurses to decrease the incidence of this problem.

Chapter 9

CARE IN NONTRADITIONAL SETTINGS

Maryanne McDonald

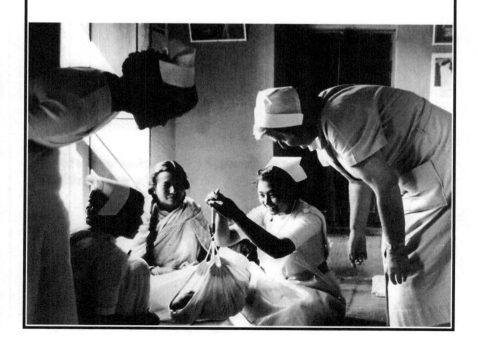

Commentary

Vernice D. Ferguson

Vulnerable populations such as the homeless present many challenges as students learn to appreciate that health status and social condition are inextricably bound. The culture of the physically disabled, with their numbers exceeding 40 million in the United States, requires greater understanding and a perspective that accommodates meeting physical and psychosocial needs as chronicity and its accommodation are better understood. Ms. McDonald describes the growth of students as they confront their own values, beliefs, biases, and prejudices in their quest to become acceptable and effective partners in care.

When Home Is a Shelter

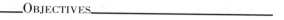

1. Initiate and apply nursing and psychosocial knowledge and skills in an unstructured environment.
2. Identify and analyze feelings, assumptions, prejudices, and biases toward culturally diverse populations.
3. Analyze and evaluate appropriate approaches to nursing assessment and the accuracy of nursing assessment.
4. Analyze and evaluate nursing interventions for appropriateness and accuracy.

You have been assigned to work in a homeless shelter for women and children. There are 10 students in your clinical group. Yours is the first group of nursing students to work at the shelter. Your assignment is to assess healthcare needs and provide healthcare at the shelter. Because this is the last semester prior to graduation, students are guided, not taught, as to what to do or how to do it. The learning process of the student is emphasized, with the goal of the administrative staff to break down the barriers to healthcare for the residents.

The homeless shelter is located in an extremely poor neighborhood. Most of the houses in the area are boarded up and empty. The shelter building is an old nursing home. Each family is assigned to one room and shares a bathroom with another family. A family consists of a mother and her children; the average number of children per mother is four. The mothers range in age from 20 to 30 years; children range from newborn to 12 years old. All of the residents are African American. All but one of the students are White.

After orientation to the shelter and meeting some of the residents, the student group meets to discuss their perceived health needs of the shelter. During the discussion, the students realize they need more information about (1) the services offered at the shelter and (2) the people living at the shelter. Their plan for the following week is to attend the morning community meeting (45 minutes) with the residents and attend teaching or therapy meetings held throughout the day.

The following week all students attended the community meeting and group sessions with the residents. The students met privately afterward to discuss their assessment. Their assessment included the following findings: approximately 30 mothers with about 60 children (younger than 5 years old) attended the community meeting. The meeting was very chaotic because of the children. The residents ran the meeting like a 12-step program, and the topics discussed at the meeting were "simple" issues like taking care of their sick children. The students felt very welcome and accepted by the residents. One of the students asked the residents what they would like the students to teach. The responses included parenting, normal child growth and development, AIDS, childhood diseases, and STDs. After discussion of their findings, some of the students wanted to begin by teaching parenting skills. Students had observed some mothers hitting their children and/or verbally abusing them. Students noticed some of the mothers spoke to their children like they were adults. However, other students felt they needed to further assess the needs of the residents before developing a plan. Students felt a more thorough assessment could be accomplished by offering a time and place for the mothers to meet with students and discuss their issues. The students also decided that half the group would attend the community meeting and half of the group would provide daycare services to the children during the community meetings.

By the third week, the students announced they would take the children to the playroom during the meeting, so the mothers could concentrate on their business. About 15 children attended the daycare. The students attending the community meeting announced they would hold an "open" teaching session from 1 to 2 P.M. Many of the residents said they would attend. The room that held the student session with residents was located on the same floor as the living quarters. The windows in the meeting room faced into the hallway, so the residents could see that the students were in the room. None of the residents came to the open session. During postconference, the students discussed their progress. They felt discouraged that no one attended the meeting. Some students felt the residents did not want to learn or improve themselves, or they would have taken advantage of the student session. After discussion, the students decided they would continue to provide daycare for the children during the community meeting (it was a much more productive meeting without the children).

By the fourth week, approximately 20 children attended the daycare with the students. During the community meeting, students announced they would have an open session for the mothers. Mothers could come and speak individually to students about any questions related to health. They also announced that the children could go to the daycare while the mothers attended the student session. Two mothers attended the meeting, stayed for five minutes, ate some food, and left. At the end of the day, students met to discuss their progress. They found that the mothers loved the daycare for children during the community meeting. The mothers who attended the afternoon open session for 5 minutes left their children in daycare for the hour. Several of the students expressed frustration and negative feelings toward the residents. They felt the mothers only stopped in at the session to eat and have someone watch their children. Other students felt they had not built a relationship with the residents or had not gained their trust. The students knocked on the residents' doors and invited them to come to the session. Other students disagreed. They felt that the residents needed to learn to take the initiative for healthcare. Once the residents left the shelter, healthcare providers would not come to their house to provide healthcare. Students questioned why the residents did not come to the session since the sessions were held several yards from the residents' rooms.

The plan for the following week was to continue with daycare, provide parenting skills during the afternoon session, and provide a five-minute in-service on parenting skills during the community meeting.

By the fifth week, 26 children attended the daycare. Students provided a 5-minute presentation on parenting skills using some examples of what they observed at the shelter. Two students shared with the residents their family history of addiction and their understanding of what some of the residents were experiencing. That afternoon, 16 mothers attended the student session. They spoke to the students in individualized sessions for 20 to 30 minutes. The students were excited with the response. They felt they were a success, not only because of the number of mothers attending the session, but because the mothers did not eat; they came only for the information.

QUESTIONS AND OBSERVATIONS

1. What were some of the factors which caused the residents' favorable response to the students?

    The residents were able to establish trust in the students. They viewed the students as sharing the same experiences as themselves (addictions) which made the students more approachable. The students demonstrated caring: playing, spending time and taking an interest in their children, and providing some food. The students were teaching a topic the residents were interested in, but the open session was too threatening. Time was an important factor. The residents had the opportunity to observe the students with their children and at community meetings.

2. What were some of the issues the students were dealing with which differed from classroom situations and other practice sites such as hospitals?

   The environment was structured in a way that was unfamiliar to the students. They did not have a captive audience. Students needed to motivate the residents to want to work with them. They were unsure of their skills. The residents were not sick; students felt there was nothing concrete (as an illness or procedure) they could work with. They needed to work with or through social issues rather than health issues; students were very task-oriented and were not always comfortable applying psychosocial skills. They felt as if they were not doing anything, needed to feel and see they accomplished something each week and this did not happen. They were learning how to work in a group in a real clinical site, not just on a classroom presentation.

3. What were some of the issues the students were dealing with on a personal level?

   The issues included prejudice toward another culture; some students were not comfortable with some of the practices of the residents. They were uncomfortable working with a population that had a different background or philosophy than the students. Many residents had lived on welfare for most of their childhood and adult lives. They were frustrated and angry that residents did not view getting a full-time job as a top priority. They were also resentful that their tax dollars were supporting people who were not interested in working. They had fears that they could experience, or had experienced, some of the things the residents had experienced: addictions, abuse, lack of support, and the judgment of others.

4. What were some of the issues of the residents?

   They did not trust healthcare providers; they had been treated badly by health professionals too many times in the past. They were afraid their questions would be perceived as "stupid." Many other issues had priority over "meeting with the students." They had a philosophy that "if you are not sick, you do not need healthcare." They did not have many experiences being with White people and were tired of being viewed as part of a group (homeless) and wanted to be seen as individuals. Privacy and confidentiality were also issues. They were not sure students did not report their problems to the shelter staff.

_____ANALYSIS AND DISCUSSION_____

This case study affected several groups of people: students, faculty, administration of the shelter, and the mothers and children of the shelter.

Students

As the weeks progressed at the shelter, it soon became apparent that the experience was more about the students than it was about the shelter residents. More time was spent on group process, discussing personal feelings, doubts, frustrations, prejudices, fears, excitement, pride, interest, volunteerism, and strengths and weakness rather than on the shelter residents.

The students' response to the shelter fell into three categories: excited to be at the shelter, did not want to be at the shelter but were receptive to learning, and did not want to be at the shelter and demonstrated negative feelings. With each succeeding group of students, it was easier for faculty to classify students into these categories and begin to work with the students at their level as early as possible during the clinical rotation. Clinical groups, in which the "excited-to-be-at-the-shelter" students took the lead, tended to stay open to the experience. The students who were more comfortable working, led at the shelter and supported the students who were having difficulty or feeling uncomfortable. Students allowed each other to express their true feelings to the group. However, students would constantly challenge and question each other regarding their beliefs, prejudice, and bias. The group worked as professionals and did not allow individual feelings to affect the work of the group. Keeping the discussion on professional issues was critical to student growth and learning. Students were not as threatened to talk about their true feelings. It appeared that if they could view their experience objectively, they could deal with negative or socially unacceptable feelings, prejudices, or beliefs. An environment was created where students could say anything and they would be accepted by other students. Students felt free to challenge each others feelings.

Clinical groups, in which the "did-not-want-to-be-at-the-shelter" students took the lead, tended to have a difficult time and many of the group members did not want to work as a group or be identified with the group.

The students who were excited to be at the shelter felt they were held back by the negative group members. Instead of accepting and challenging the negative group members, students tried to convince them that they were wrong. The negative students made issues personal and were not always able to express or resolve the problem as professionals. This did not work. There was little or no common ground for the students to work on. Eventually, students worked around negative group members. It was much easier for the "excited student" leaders to motivate the "negative" students.

Overall, students felt the clinical experience was very beneficial. Some of their comments were: "I grew in ways I never knew I could"; "It was tough working with some students but it forced me to use skills and talents I never knew I had . . . I never realized I was a leader"; "I did not realize how judgmental I was . . . I thought I would always be caring but I realized I sometimes care only if the person meets my expectations as a person"; "I was shocked by some of the practices of the residents, for example, never having a job, but after spending time with residents and getting to know them personally, I realize they never had the opportunity or the know-how . . . how could they know if their parents never had a job either?"; "I used to get mad when I would be doing discharge teaching in the hospital for a homeless mother and she would only be half listening . . . now I know why."

Students needed time to think and process their feelings and beliefs. Many students did not realize their prejudices or biases until they were forced to face them at the shelter. Students found it difficult to keep their former beliefs when they worked with residents at the shelter. Personal experiences changed them. They began to see more commonalties than differences as they listened and worked with residents.

Although it took most of the seven-week rotation, students realized the most important intervention they provided at the shelter was their presence. Residents and shelter staff said over and over again, that just being at the shelter was instrumental in changing how the residents viewed health professionals. By the end of the rotation, approximately 90 percent of the students enjoyed the experience and felt they had learned and grown. Ten percent said they "got through the rotation."

Faculty

Providing a nonjudgmental and supportive environment allowed students to take responsibility for their beliefs and an opportunity to change or expand them. The intent of this clinical rotation was to provide students with an opportunity to apply their knowledge and skills; process was emphasized over outcome. Faculty were considered facilitators and not instructors. Initially, students wanted more structure or to be told what to do. Once they realized this was not going to happen they assumed responsibility. Students stopped trying to do what they thought faculty wanted and worked on what they wanted to do. This allowed students to act as they truly felt and brought controversial issues to the discussion. Students depended on each other to accomplish their work. They realized the outcome was a result of their work alone. They, rather than the faculty, challenged each other to deal with their own issues, so they could be productive as a group. Students generally provided a nonjudgmental and supportive environment for each other.

Administration of the Shelter

Staff at the shelter did not have established expectations of the students. Since it was a new program, students were free to develop their own program. However, staff did not want students to provide primary healthcare at the shelter. The staff wanted the residents to develop the skills of obtaining healthcare in the community, as they would when they left the shelter. This allowed the students to become less focused on tasks and more focused on process.

Residents

When asked, the residents felt the most important intervention by the students was "them just being here . . . that shows they care about us." Residents seemed to learn most from students' examples rather than teaching sessions. Comments from the residents included: "I saw how all the kids would run up and hug the students when they came into the shelter . . . jumping up and down . . . I realized my kids never ran and hugged me, so I started watching what the students did so I could do it too"; "They never judged us . . . always showed me respect"; "I realized not all nurses are the same, there are some really nice nurses"; "I am going to nursing school!"

Cultural barriers were broken down for both the students and the residents.

_____ANNOTATED REFERENCES_____

Burg, M. A. (1994). Health problems of sheltered homeless women and their dependent children. *Health and Social Work, 19*(2), 125–131.

This article provides the student with a general knowledge of the health and social problems of homeless women and children. The article demonstrates the fact that health problems go hand-in-hand with social problems; a health professional can not address health problems without addressing social problems.

Davidhizar, R., & Frank, B. (1992). Understanding the physical and psychosocial stressors of the child who is homeless. *Pediatric Nursing, 18*(6), 559–562.

This article offers a unique and realistic view of the child's perspective toward homelessness. The child is often the most overlooked segment of the homeless population. This article emphasizes the need to address the issues of the homeless children to prevent the child from becoming a homeless adult.

Eddins, E. (1993, Spring). Characteristics, health status and service needs of sheltered homeless families. *The ABNF Journal*, 440–444.

This article provides a comprehensive perspective on the type of services needed by homeless families. The needs of homeless families are unique and different from the need of a single homeless person. The similar characteristics found in this population will guide the students in their assessment and plan for health services.

Norton, D., & Ridemour, N. (1995). Homeless women and children: The challenge of health promotion. *Nurse Practitioner Forum, 6*(1), 29–33.

This article provides perspective on the difficulty of health promotion to homeless women and children. The difficulties of initiating health promotion to a population whose main concerns are food, shelter, and clothing are discussed. The article provides the student with the information to use to motivate homeless women and children.

Scholler-Jacquish, A. (1996). RN to BSN students in a walk-in health clinic for the homeless. *N & NC: Perspectives on Community, 17*(3), 118–123.

The wide range of health and social problems of the homeless are discussed, as well as methods to address these issues. The article is an excellent example of the issues a student needs to address before providing healthcare to this population.

Traumatic, Life-Altering Experience

──────────────OBJECTIVES──────────────

1. Reflect and discuss his or her values and beliefs related to caring for someone whose lifestyle has caused their own disability.
2. Identify common assumptions made by health professionals when caring for someone from a different culture and/or community.
3. Analyze the role of the nurse in planning, implementing, and evaluating care for someone from a different culture.

*M*r. G. is a 32-year-old male. He has just been discharged from the hospital after four months. He is a quadriplegic post trauma. Mr. G. is staying with one of his four sisters. His sister is 34 years old with two children, 6 and 13 years old. The primary home health nurse has asked you to visit Mr. G. This will be the second home health visit since his discharge from the hospital four days ago. The primary nurse provides some background information.

Mr. G. was injured in a fight on the corner of his street. Though no one witnessed the fight, drugs were suspected to be the cause of the fight. Mr. G. has a long-standing history of drug abuse. He has never been able to find work. During his hospitalization, his family rarely visited him. When the nurses asked his family to come to the hospital to learn how to care for him, they frequently missed appointments. When they did come to the hospital, the staff reported the family seemed inattentive to instruction. Mr. G. was discharged from the hospital to home.

Medical Orders:

–Isocal 250 ccs every 4 hours.
–quad cough every 2 hours.
–fluid intake 2000 cc/day.
–bowel program.

When you visit Mr. G. at 10 A.M., you knock on the door for almost 15 minutes before his sister answers the door. His sister, K. states she thought you were the church people and that is why she did not open the door. You walk into the dining room where Mr. G. is lying on the bed. Your assessment findings include the following:

—rails at both bases.
—temperature is 101 degrees orally.
—vital signs: 102/70, 96, 30.
—urine output: 400 ccs last 24 hours.
quad cough every 2 hours while in bed.

You ask K. when is the last time she performed the quad cough on Mr. G. She responds "yesterday" and begins to put on her coat to go out to the store.

———————————QUESTIONS AND OBSERVATIONS———————————

1. Why is K. behaving as she is?

    Students usually respond that K. is noncompliant and does not really want to take care of her brother. When asked to explain, students will list behaviors such as not visiting Mr. G. in the hospital, taking so long to answer the door, and an obvious lack of care (based on home assessment).
2. Ask students to list all the reasons, other than noncompliance, why K. may be acting this way.

    She may feel overwhelmed, or "stupid" in front of health professionals and is afraid to ask questions and that is why she stopped visiting him in the hospital. She is afraid to care for Mr. G. for fear she may hurt him. She does not want to take care of Mr. G., but no one in the home wants to do it. She is resentful toward her brother, who has been a problem all his life and now she has to "pay for his behavior." She does not know where to begin to care for him for there is so much to do.
3. Why does the home health nurse need to be concerned about K.?
4. During your one-hour visit, what would you teach K.?
5. Keeping in mind that you do not want to overwhelm K. any further, what teaching strategies would you use?
6. What additional resources would you use?

———————————ANALYSIS AND DISCUSSION———————————

Reinforce with students the need to look beyond what they would consider "noncompliance" and identify other reasons why a caregiver may be nonsupportive. This can be done over a number of visits to the home. First, a trusting relationship needs to be developed. K. needs to feel she can say anything to you and you will not judge but support her. Students may continue to feel judgmental toward K. With guided discussion, they realize that if they do not work with K. and resolve her problems, they cannot help Mr. G. Mr. G.'s welfare depends on K. In home health, the home health nurse needs to work with what and who is available and obtain support from the primary caregiver. Health professionals are not available 24 hours a day as they are in the hospital. Also, in home health, the caregivers are "in control" rather than the nurse. The home health nurse needs to be able to motivate the client/caregiver to change behavior. (Being judgmental does not motivate anyone.)

Students need to prioritize what needs to be taught first. They tend to want to teach everything. In view of K. feeling overwhelmed, teaching more than one procedure may frustrate K. even further. Students can teach through role modeling and asking K.'s assistance while the student works with the patient. For example, offer the patient sips of water throughout the whole visit. Teach the nieces and nephews to offer water to their uncle each time they pass through the dining room. Role modeling is less threatening than teaching K. and asking her to demonstrate. Spending time with K. at the beginning of each visit and asking her how she is managing and praising her work will provide support to K.

With Mr. G.'s inability to work, he is probably on medical assistance. His home care benefit is limited. However, there are many community resources available. The student can contact the following (1) social worker at a rehabilitation center to identify services and resources, (2) legislative office in the community, (3) vocational technical school, and (4) city and state services department.

_____ANNOTATED REFERENCES_____

Leininger, M. M. (1991). *Culture care diversity and universality: A theory of nursing.* New York: NLN Press.

This publication provides the student with a framework for the assessment, planning, implementation, and evaluation of health care to diverse populations. It provides a comprehensive approach to cultural assessment.

Spradley, B. (Ed.). (1991). *Readings in community health nursing* (4th ed.). Philadelphia: Lippincott.

Maryanne McDonald

This text provides classical articles related to healthcare issues in both public health and community health. The text addresses community at the client level as well as at the community and public health levels. While it is written for the discipline of nursing, it is an appropriate text for any discipline. One section of the text, 10 chapters, is dedicated to the cultural dimension of community health nursing, offering the student a broad range of the cultural dimensions that need to be addressed in a community assessment.

Chapter 10

PROBLEM-FOCUSED CARE

JoAnne Reifsnyder

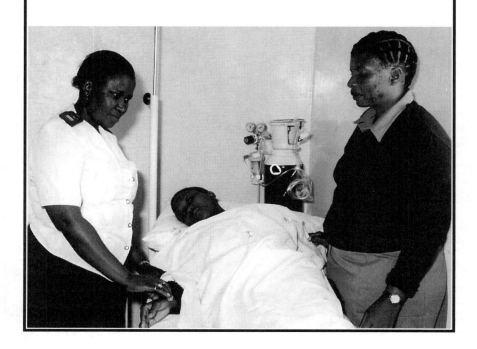

COMMENTARY

Vernice D. Ferguson

The case studies presented by Ms. Reifsnyder demonstrate the importance of problem identification. The critical role of the nurse as an advocate comes into full play as Mr. Y.'s care is managed and the older adults in an urban complex accommodated.

The case of Mr. Y. illustrates the need to give attention to cultural values as better understanding of the person's coping mechanisms emerge. The danger of labeling behaviors, noncompliance, for instance, must be guarded against by care providers. By identifying the values that guide the behavior of those served the care provider can effect acceptable and effective care.

Fostering aggregate assessments by groups of students enrich the problem-solving process as creativity is fostered.

When Old World Meets New

1. Reflect on her or his values that underlie assumptions made about caring for older adults.
2. List and discuss reasons why older individuals may stop taking medications.
3. Analyze the role of the nurse in caring for an individual who is unwilling/unable to share details of his history during the interview.

*A*n elderly Chinese gentleman, G. Y., first visited the health office at an urban multipurpose senior center for a blood pressure screening. Mr. Y.'s blood pressure reading was extremely high in both arms, with minimal difference between right and left readings or sitting and standing readings. Mr. Y. has an obvious left-sided hemiparesis. He understood and responded appropriately to questions, but his speech was slow and dysarthric. Mr. Y. lived alone in a small apartment in the city's Chinatown section. He denied current health problems and stated that he took prescription medication for his blood pressure as directed.

Mr. Y. stated that he shopped for and prepared his meals, but indicated that he could only carry small bundles due to his left-sided paralysis. He used the city's subsidized transportation for the elderly and disabled whenever possible, but occasionally had to use taxi service when other transport was not available. He walked from his apartment to nearby stores to do his food shopping. Mr. Y. was covered both by Medicare and medical assistance, so his prescription medications required only a small co-payment. Mr. Y. lived on a small fixed income. He had no family in the United States and gave his landlord's name and telephone number as an emergency contact. Mr. Y. visited the senior center three times weekly, during which time he ate lunch and sat in one of the lounge areas. He had not formed any friendships with other seniors at the center, and smiled and shook his head "no" when questioned about aspects of his life that were most important to him. Mr. Y. was reluctant to give the name of his physician and was resistant to the nurse's encouragement to consult his physician about the elevated blood pressure.

The nurse concluded the interview by expressing concern over Mr. Y.'s blood pressure, and once again queried him about his blood pressure medication. He did not have the prescription with him. The nurse told Mr. Y. that sometimes people took fewer of their pills than prescribed, or stopped taking the pills all together for a variety of reasons. She listed some of the reasons, and asked Mr. Y. if any of these might be true for him. Mr. Y. reluctantly stated that he was almost out of pills, but was making them last by taking them only every other day rather than twice daily. The nurse offered to assist Mr. Y. by telephoning his physician for a renewal or scheduling an appointment, if necessary. Mr. Y. firmly shook his head "no."

When approximately one half hour had elapsed since the beginning of the interview, the nurse stated to Mr. Y. "I am concerned about your blood pressure, but I'm not sure how to help you. Is there anything that I can do to help you?" Mr. Y. hesitated, then revealed that he "did not like" his doctor and was convinced that his doctor did not like him either. He adamantly stated that he would not go back to that doctor, and asked the nurse if she could find him someone else. Mr. Y. refused to share any further details about his relationship with his current doctor, and repeated his previous statements of his wishes. The nurse assured Mr. Y. that she would help him with this. Mr. Y. agreed to show the nurse his medical assistance wallet information, which gave the name of his "primary" physician and a telephone number for the medical assistance office. After assessing Mr. Y.'s preference for physician location and hospital affiliation, the nurse offered to make the necessary telephone calls to secure the change in physician. With Mr. Y.'s permission, a same-day appointment with a nurse practitioner in the new physician's office was made, a summary of the nurse's assessment was communicated to the nurse practitioner in the office, and transportation was arranged both to the physician's office and home from the office. Because the client had been assigned to his former physician through the medical assistance program, multiple telephone calls were required to effect a change for the client. The combination of the client's speech difficulty and his lack of ready access to a telephone had presented a significant barrier to his ability to self-manage his health status. Consequently, he coped the only way he knew how.

QUESTIONS

---

1. How should the nurse proceed with an interview when the client is reluctant to share his relevant history? Identify at least three options.

2. Select the one "best" option and discuss the rationale for your selection. Does everyone in the group agree? Analyze the areas of agreement and disagreement in your group. How would you characterize them?

3. What is the nurse's priority in the continued interview with Mr. Y.? What further assessment should the nurse conduct?

4. Make a list of reasons why people do not take medications as prescribed. How could you classify these reasons (i.e., are some reasons relevant only to a particular group, are there underlying commonalities such as financial constraints)?

5. Discuss strategies for intervention within each category of reasons. What are the implications for community/ public/ home health nurses? For hospital-based nurses?

6. Why might Mr. Y. be reluctant to contact his physician or to have the nurse do so? What are the underlying values associated with reasons that your group has identified?

7. What were the keys to the success of the nurse's intervention with Mr. Y.? How should the nurse evaluate the outcome of the interventions? What additional issues should the nurse address with Mr. Y. on subsequent visits to the health office?

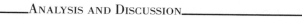

ANALYSIS AND DISCUSSION

Effective nursing care depends to a great extent on the quality of the relationship that the nurse establishes with the client. The effective nurse-client relationship is built on trust, openness, and acceptance of the individual's unique beliefs and behaviors. Acceptance of client behaviors rests upon the nurse's ability to identify the client's values, analyze the impact of these on the client's health and well-being, and accept that his or her own values are not the standards by which clients should live.

In Mr. Y.'s case, the client's behavior (decreasing his dose of blood pressure medication to make it last longer) provides a clue to his underlying values. A "value" is a standard or quality that is considered important to an individual (Fry, 1994). An individual holds many values, and these are typically organized mentally into a hierarchy. That is, a person may value both honesty and protection of loved ones from harm. For that individual, one value will need to be placed above the other when action is required, such as the honest telling of bad news that may devastate the person receiving it. The way in which values are organized is highly individual.

Values conflicts may occur within the individual, as described above, or they may occur between individuals. For example, Mr. Y. clearly placed values regarding his integrity as a person and avoidance of unsatisfactory relationships with others above his own physical health. The nurse who interviews Mr. Y. may subscribe to the belief that clients are responsible for the physical health above some (or all) other needs. Often when we label clients such as Mr. Y. "noncompliant," what we mean is that their "noncompliant" behavior is not consistent with the values of healthcare providers. It is sometimes difficult for us to understand why or how a client like Mr. Y. could put other needs first, given the serious consequences that may result from untreated hypertension.

Culturally sensitive care demands that healthcare providers obtain an adequate history, through which they identify the values that guide the patient's behavior. The culturally competent nurse assists the client to clarify values and make choices that are consistent with those values. To do this, the nurse must be aware of her or his own values and be comfortable when clients' choices and behaviors are other than what the nurse would choose for her or himself. Culturally sensitive care can occur only when the nurse acts on information supplied by the client—not on assumptions about the individual, the individual's ethnic background or other characteristics.

Obtaining an adequate history from a client takes time. A reality of today's healthcare settings is that time is at a premium. Therefore, the nurse must be able to quickly assess what the client's most immediate needs are and respond to them. Mr. Y.'s case illustrates how complex some client problems can be. Had the nurse decided to discontinue the interview at an earlier point, she would have missed what the essential problem actually was. In this case, Mr. Y.'s uncontrolled hypertension was a symptom of another unmet need. Had the nurse responded simply to the hypertension—by instructing Mr. Y. about taking his medications correctly, talking with him about the problems that can result from untreated hypertension, or even calling his physician—she would have ended the encounter with a very false sense of security. The time taken to interview this client was well spent, as the root problem was not revealed until quite late in the process.

Clients vary widely in their abilities and/or willingness to follow prescribed treatment regimens. It is essential to effective nursing care that the nurse possess knowledge of common problems that older people encounter when taking medications. Although medication mismanagement is one area in which nurses may label patients noncompliant, such a label speaks more about the nurse's assumptions than it does about the client's actual problem. Nurses may mistakenly assume that the client who has been taught about medication management should be able to follow the regimen without problems, or may mistakenly conclude the client's problem is a continued knowledge deficit. In fact, many older clients may stop or reduce their medications due to unpleasant side effects, financial concerns, or other problems (Ebersole & Hess, 1994). An effective strategy that the nurse can use to apply such knowledge of older people is to phrase questions in such a way as to make it "okay" for the client to admit that his self-administration of medications has varied from the original recommendation. For example, the nurse can say, "Many people find it difficult to take their medications exactly as they were prescribed. Do you ever miss a dose?" Clients who trust that they will not be judged for their choices are far more likely to share information about those choices.

ANNOTATED REFERENCES

Ebersole, P., & Hess, P. (1994). *Toward healthy aging*. Philadelphia: Mosby.

This is a classic text for teaching principles of nursing the older adult. It addresses some of the particularly challenging issues of caring for the elderly in community settings, such as medication management, elder abuse, and socioeconomic disparities.

Fry, S. T. (1994). *Ethics in nursing practice: A guide to ethical decision making*. Geneva, Switzerland: International Council of Nurses.

The author worked with the Professional Services Committee of the ICN to prepare this guidebook for nurses' ethical decision making. It takes a unique approach in that cases are deliberately constructed for relevance to nurses practicing in diverse international settings. Parts I and II of the text present fundamental concepts enhanced by lucid examples and applications. In Part III the author applies the content to critical issues in nursing practice. The presentation of the concepts and the use of examples, case studies, and questions for discussion with analyses make this book especially useful in teaching nursing ethics to students and practicing nurses alike.

New Places, New Faces

1. Identify advantages and disadvantages to assessment and intervention at the level of the aggregate.
2. Suggest health-related issues that could be addressed in a community of older adults living in an urban apartment complex.
3. Apply the nursing process to the care of groups or aggregates in the community.

*S*tudents who were completing a community health clinical rotation were assigned to a high-rise apartment building for the elderly and disabled. The building is located in an urban area and houses several hundred residents. Students made home visits to self-identified and social worker-identified residents for health promotion/disease prevention and for chronic illness management. In conferencing after visits, students compared their experiences and identified that residents frequently described unhealthy eating habits, most notably the inclusion of greater than recommended amounts of sodium and saturated fat. Residents in this building tended not to socialize with other residents, and the building did not include a common area for sharing meals.

The students conducted a target group assessment to determine whether the residents demonstrated trends that could be addressed by an aggregate approach. A variety of data sources were sampled, including city census track data, morbidity and mortality data, building-specific demographic data, key informant interviews, door to door surveys, and a walking survey of the surrounding area. Students analyzed the data, and concluded that lack of access to convenient and affordable food shopping was a fundamental variable contributing to observed unhealthy eating habits.

The students in this case determined that residents would be very interested in availing themselves of a weekly bus to a shopping center that was approximately 20 blocks away, if such service were available. Public buses were already available, but not suited to the residents' physical frailty and need for assistance in carrying/stowing purchases. The students contacted the owner of the shopping center to assess his interest, drafted a proposal for bus service subsidized by a combination of store owners' contribution and a small fare, then organized a meeting of key individuals. The students were not able to bring this project to a close during their community health experience, but they made arrangements for follow-up by others.

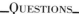

QUESTIONS

1. What organizing framework could guide your data collection when assessing a target group or community? Compare and contrast several approaches. What criteria would you use for selecting a particular framework?
2. Is the target group that was assessed in this example a "community"? Why or why not?
3. What additional data would you collect? Why?
4. State a nursing diagnosis for the target group, and suggest three approaches to intervention. Which one would you choose? What is your rationale?
5. What criteria would you apply to evaluate the outcome of the intervention that you selected?

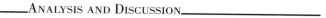

ANALYSIS AND DISCUSSION

Assessment of a group or aggregate involves similar aims and processes as assessment of an individual or family. The advantages to assessment and intervention at the level of the aggregate may be less clear. In the case example, student nurses had formed relationships with various clients living in the same apartment building. Many identified nutrition as an area in which intervention was called for. The students could have worked in isolation, addressing each individual client's needs. Each client would have participated in a plan of care designed to meet his or her unique needs, and each presumably would have realized some positive outcomes that were jointly specified by the client and the nurse. Such a situation mirrors what regularly does happen in healthcare—multiple providers in the same geographic area addressing similar needs with individual clients.

Aggregate assessment of older adults in this case example has the advantage of optimally utilizing the healthcare provider's resources. When a problem or health care need is identified in each of a number of individuals, a trend often emerges that was not evident until the data was examined as a whole. This phenomenon of stepping back from the trees in order to see the forest is a cornerstone to holistic care of the individual. Nurses who focus beyond any singular aspect of an individual client during assessment, such as a physical symptom of an illness, will see the significance of the broader picture, which includes the interplay of multiple variables. Similarly, on the aggregate level, the nurse who assesses many individuals in a larger group will be able to see the significance of the broader health picture of a community. As nurses strive to move healthcare into a more proactive, preventive system of care extending beyond the limited illness focus, it is especially important that they begin to look at the trends in larger groups and design interventions to reach them. An expansion of nursing's sphere of influence and an enhanced impact on the health of the nation as a whole will result.

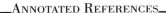

ANNOTATED REFERENCES

Lubkin, I. M. (1990). *Chronic illness: impact and interventions* (2nd ed.). Boston: Jones and Bartlett.

This important text provides a foundation for teaching restorative nursing. The author addresses key issues in chronic illness management, and provides an unusually clear conception of the nursing care that is relevant to chronically ill individuals.

Spradley, B. W. (1991). *Readings in community health nursing* (4th ed.). Philadelphia: Lippincott.

This text is a compilation of papers on a variety of topics in community health nursing. The book is divided into eight parts, each emphasizing a different aspect of community health nursing practice. In addition to sections devoted to classical concepts in community health nursing, the book contains a section on cultural dimensions and a final section that addresses politics and change agents.

Chapter 11

MINIMIZING COMMUNICATION BARRIERS

June Stewart

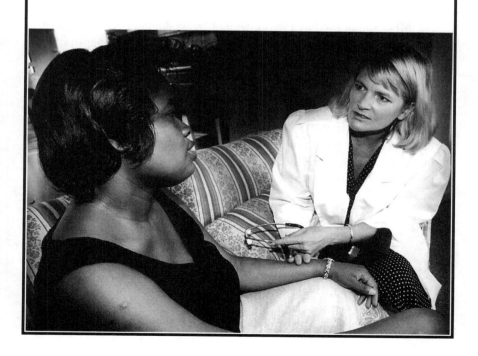

COMMENTARY

Vernice D. Ferguson

Respect demonstrated between care providers is as important as respect accorded care recipients. Dr. Stewart addresses this need in the first case study. Hierarchical positioning rather than team relationships in an organization can thwart gathering useful information that can improve the care provided to people. Capitalizing on the information that the African American employee could provide—in this case, whether she is or is not another professional nurse—would have lent useful insight since she comes from a similar cultural background.

Among the important lessons learned during the stormy 1960s in the United States, as African Americans sought equality in treatment and opportunity, was this: look to the people who are experiencing the problems to seek remedies for them. Miss P. would have done well to have considered this strategy.

In the second case study, Mrs. Simon's daughter, a journalist, graphically describes the many affronts which her old and ailing mother experienced in one of America's best hospitals as care was provided.

Mrs. Simon died at age 85. One of the last sentences she spoke before she died was, "my name is Mrs. Simon." During this hospitalization she was referred to as "Doll," "Grannie," or "Auntie." Mrs. Simon's daughter reminds us that her mother's first name was Anna and that she came from a fairly formal European background in which older people are rarely on a first-name basis with anyone except relatives and close friends.

In a culture where informality tends to be the norm, we must remind ourselves continually that we must ask those whom we serve and those that we work with how they wish to be addressed.

Elliott, E. (1984). My name is Mrs. Simon. *Ladies Home Journal,* August. pp 18–19, 150.

You Don't Know Me

—————————OBJECTIVES—————————

1. Identify barriers to effective communication between and among ethnically diverse care givers.
2. Cite examples of physiological variables that can provide a basis for decision making in ethnically diverse healthcare settings.
3. Explore methodologies that could be utilized in nursing programs to address the requisite knowledge and skills necessary to deliver safe, effective culturally competent nursing care.

Mrs. G. is a 54-year-old African American who is employed at a well baby clinic. Miss P., a 33-year-old Caucasian pediatric nurse practitioner, is in charge of the clinic. While performing a routine assessment on a 4-month-old African American infant both Mrs. G. and Miss P. noticed what appeared to be bruises on the infant's sacral area. Miss P. immediately suspected child abuse and quickly decided that her suspicions were justified and must be reported to the appropriate authorities. Mrs. G., somewhat annoyed by what she perceived to be a "too-quick-to-come-to-decision" attitude on the part of Miss P., suggested that the observations first should be discussed with the mother of the infant adding that "these kind of marks are not uncommon in African American as well as Asian and Latin infants." Miss P. responded, "Well, I have never heard that before. You are probably trying to cover up for your people." Mrs. G.'s response was to promptly and angrily walk out of the examining room, slamming the door.

—————————QUESTIONS—————————

1. What factors could have made Miss P. conclude that the infant was probably a victim of child abuse?

2. What factors could have caused Mrs. G. to suggest they talk to the mother before acting hastily?
3. Did either nurse act inappropriately?
4. What do you think precipitated Mrs. G.'s reaction?
5. What actions on the part of Miss P. and Mrs. G. might have led to a better understanding of how mutual respect among healthcare providers can enhance the effectiveness of providing care to culturally diverse clients?

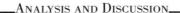

ANALYSIS AND DISCUSSION

Mrs. G. is a minority among minorities. According to Greer (1995), African Americans and other minorities comprise only 9.8 percent of the total number of registered nurses in the United States. Miss P. is providing care for clients, the majority of whom are from ethnic backgrounds different than hers.

Both nurses are concerned about the provision of care and protecting the welfare of their clients. Miss P.'s response represents direct concern about the welfare of her client. Mrs. G. also shares the same concern but indicates a desire to gather more information about the dynamics of the family of which the client is a member. Mrs. G. also apparently was familiar with what probably could have been a causative factor of the infant's condition. Miss P. missed an opportunity to demonstrate respect for Mrs. G.'s knowledge, and what could have been an educational experience of benefit to the well baby clinic as a whole: providing culture-specific information for future assessment of clients.

Lea (1994) argues that nurses need to consider the different ethnic and cultural backgrounds of their patients in order to provide effective and safe nursing care. Mrs. G. and Miss P. could function effectively as a team in providing culturally competent care if they were able to identify the causation of their actions.

Miss P. could have elicited more information from Mrs. G. and other sources but appeared to dismiss the information given as insignificant because she had never heard of it and placed Mrs. G. in a defensive stance by accusing or at least implying that Mrs. G. was "covering up for your people."

Mrs. G. acted improperly when she removed herself in an unprofessional manner. An understanding or at least a recognition of culturally sensitive issues is warranted by both nurses.

————————————————ANNOTATED REFERENCES————————————————

Greer, D. B. (1995, March-April). Minority underrepresentation in nursing: socioeconomic and political effects. *ABNF Journal, 6*(2), 44–46.

This article discusses the under representation of minorities in nursing; the effect that this under representation can have on patient outcomes, and possible
solutions.

Lea, A. (1994, August). Nursing in today's multicultural society: a transcultural
   perspective. *Journal of Advanced Nursing, 20*(2), 307–313.

Lea argues that safe effective nursing care cannot be given without an awareness
of ethnic and cultural differences.

Price, J. C., & Cordell, B. (1994). Cultural diversity and patient teaching. *Journal of Continuing Education in Nursing, 25*(4), 163–166.

Cordell and Price present a strong argument for the understanding of cultural diversity and how this understanding can impact on effective outcomes and compliance in patients.

On My Own

1. Explore cultural and racial sensitivity that can impact on the client's health seeking behaviors.
2. Identify cultural norms and traditions in order to gain a perspective on personal values and similarities and differences among individuals and groups.
3. Explore sociocultural and historical perspectives that can impact on the dignity of clients.

*M*rs. J. is a 92-year-old African American widow who has lived alone and maintained her small suburban home since the death of her husband 20 years ago. Mrs. J., a former educator, maintains membership in several professional organizations and takes great pride in the fact that "I am the oldest member of my sorority who still goes to the convention every year."

She enjoys gardening, reading, sewing, and cooking. Although Mrs. J. considers herself to be in good health and mentally sound, she is concerned that she "forgets sometimes." It is the "forgetting sometimes" that concerns her children. According to her 60-year-old daughter, "Mother starts to cook and forgets that the stove is on and has had several small kitchen fires as a result." On one occasion, Mrs. J. fell asleep and woke up to a house full of smoke and the smoke alarm blaring loudly. Fortunately, a neighbor who was planting flowers heard the alarm and, after it did not go off, went to check on Mrs. J. Although there were no injuries and minimal property damage, the neighbor contacted one of Mrs. J.'s children. This last incident left Mrs. J.'s children concerned about her safety. Although her son checks her daily, the family felt that they needed to seek professional advice that would assist family members in determining what means were available to provide a safe, independent environment for their mother.

A family friend suggested that they contact the community health association in order to "find out what is available." Mrs. J.'s family requested her permission to make the initial investigation and Mrs. J. reluctantly agreed, although she did not see the necessity.

Upon contacting the agency, it was agreed that a nurse would be sent to the home to make an assessment of Mrs. J.'s status. The nurse assigned to the case was a 23-year-old White female who, upon arriving at the home of Mrs. J., rang the doorbell which was promptly and cheerfully answered by Mrs. J. The nurse introduced herself in her usually cheerful manner, "Hi, I'm Ginny; you are Helen?" Mrs. J. responded, "Good afternoon, I am Mrs. J." Mrs. J. appeared to be angry and irritated which interfered with the ability to communicate effectively. The nurse said, "Helen, you appear to be upset." Mrs. J. replied, "Yes, I am very upset. I do not recall giving you permission to call me by my first name, and I consider it to be an insult that you assumed this behavior to be acceptable."

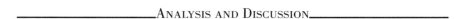

QUESTIONS

1. What assumptions did the nurse make when addressing Mrs. J.?
2. What factors could have accounted for Mrs. J.'s anger?
3. How can cultural norms be utilized effectively in establishing a nurse-client relationship?
4. Did the nurse demonstrate knowledge necessary or the acquisition of requested knowledge to deliver safe, competent, culturally sensitive care?

ANALYSIS AND DISCUSSION

Although Mrs. J. agreed to allow her family to investigate resources to assist her, she did so reluctantly. Her reluctance could have stemmed from her independent lifestyle and any intrusion on that lifestyle could have been perceived as a loss of independence. Conversely, African American elderly often look to the family to make health and safety related decisions and accept suggestions presented even if reluctant to do so.

The concern of her children about her safety was justified. She was at risk for bodily harm related to an accidental fire. Mrs. J.'s reaction probably could have been positive if the nurse had demonstrated an awareness of the appropriate cultural norms and taboos when addressing an elderly African American. The use of a first name by a younger person is considered to be rude. The assumption of permission to use one's first name by a young, white person is not only perceived as rude but also seen as a blatant lack of respect. Further, it elicits previously negative experiences of racial description in which African Americans were automatically addressed by first names in order to denote a superior-inferior relationship.

In community-based nursing, the nurse must be keenly aware of the norms and values of clients. This awareness becomes even more important when the nurse is a guest in a client's home. According to Capers (1992), it is in the community and home that cultural lifeways become more apparent to the healthcare provider. Culture cannot be separated from the nurse's interaction with the client. Mrs. J.'s response to the nurse's introduction represented a perceived lack of respect, an attitude of superiority on the part of the nurse, and a loss of dignity and independence.

ANNOTATED REFERENCES

Capers, C. F. (1992). Teaching cultural content: A nursing education imperative. *Holistic Nursing Practice, 6*(3), 19–28.

The author presents the role of nurse educators who are preparing their students to be culturally competent. Explores curriculum, approaches, and content.

Nance, T. A. (1995). Intercultural communication: Finding common ground. *J.O.G.N.N., 24*(3), 249–255.

The author addresses the significance of understanding cultural differences and similarities in communication and the critical nature of similarity.

Chapter 12

TAKING CONTROL

Dolores Patrinos

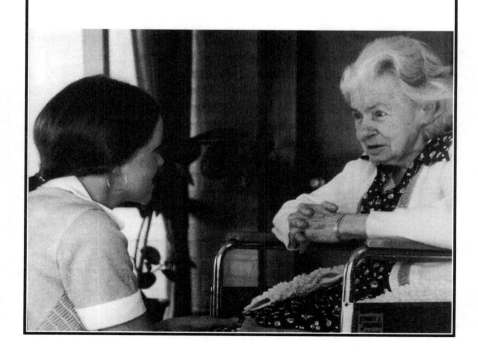

Vernice D. Ferguson

Cultural barriers thwart the ability of marginalized people to take control of their lives. Ms. Patrinos uses this case study to address the strategies that the transformational nurse can use as the voices of the unheard become heard.

If They Can't Help Me,
I Don't Need Them

———————————————————OBJECTIVES———————————————————

1. To examine the narrative as a therapeutic conversation for problem definition and problem solving.
2. To analyze how cultural barriers serve to quiet the voices of poor and minority females in single family households.
3. To critique the strategies used by the transformational nurse as women come out of the shadow and enter into the dialogic space for empowerment purposes.

*M*s. J. is a 27-year-old African American, single parent who is seven months pregnant. She has three other children—11 and 5-year-old twins. The nurse first met Ms. J. when she brought her son, Theodore, to the Crisis center to seek help "with his stealing, truancy, using drugs, and being abusive to his sisters."

Ms. J. had already approached several agencies seeking assistance with her son's behavioral problems. None of these efforts had resulted in "any real help." According to Ms. J., "they asked me a lot of questions and wrote reports. Then when I finally thought I would get some help for Theodore, the man (referring to the psychologist) just played some games with him."

Ms. J.'s affect is sad and she presents a mood of helplessness while talking about her life. She is the second generation experiencing the cycle of poverty, having left school in the eleventh grade during her first pregnancy. When discussing her family of origin, Ms. J. states that her mother is deceased and her father has been "out of the picture for a long time" due to alcoholism. She has three brothers, all of whom she describes as substance abusers. One is presently incarcerated. She has one sister who "lives thousands of miles away."

Ms. J. and her children live in a rented three-bedroom house. She receives Aid to Families with Dependent Children. She tells the nurse about two significant relationships with men over the past 12 years. The first relationship lasted for 6 years and produced her first three children. Her last relationship extended over 5 years. During a part of that period her partner was in prison for legal problems related to drug use. The relationship terminated during the first trimester of the present pregnancy. The men in her life are perceived as marginal to her existence, and she states, "if they can't help me, I don't need them."

She confides that she had "watched out for whether she would get pregnant" and felt very sad and dejected when she discovered that she had failed to prevent this pregnancy. She hopes to have a tubal ligation after delivery since nothing else has worked for her. She has made one prenatal visit to a local hospital but has not discussed her plans with anyone "as yet." Presently, she plans to give up the infant for adoption as soon as it is born.

Ms. J. describes her health status as "tired all the time." She spends a great deal of time in bed. She seeks medical attention at the nearest emergency room of her home. Her children's activities outside of school center on playing outdoors near the house until about ten o'clock in the evening. The family does not belong to any formal religious community but Ms. J. believes in God and prays since she is too tired to attend church.

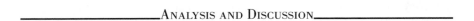

QUESTIONS

1. What are the challenges in this family to the nurse socialized in the reality of the dominant culture?
2. What are the opportunities to provide holistic care to this family?
3. How can the nurse develop skills in learning to hear the multiple voices of women in families?

ANALYSIS AND DISCUSSION

The healing potential of the narrative through which the multiple voices of women are heard for problem definition and problem solving lend an insightful dimension as care is provided. The nursing literature sensitive to narrative also describes a paradigm shift in nursing practice. That shift assumes human experiences are created and interpreted as part of the context in which they take place (Clarke & Cody, 1994). The practice of professional nursing at the end of the 20th century in America occurs in varied environments inhabited by people from various ethnic groups, molded by gender expectations, and class and race politics (Marable, 1995). By implication, there are multiple worldviews that make up the totality of human experiences. In addition, some authors believe that "socially responsible" nursing care means supporting the development of interpersonal networks of family, friends, and neighbors for life sustaining purposes (Bridges & Lyman, 1993; West, 1994). The paradigm shift is about nurses making connections with and understanding the worldviews of those we define as clients.

The paradigm shift for nursing practice also alters the form and content for nursing education. In our diverse society, students need to learn how to listen to the multiple voices of clients. A person's voice is a methodology through which a sense of identity is expressed. This identity is an evolving sense of who one is, what one thinks, feels, knows, believes, and cares about (Weingarten, 1994). The voices tell about a woman's experience as an individual, wife, mother, daughter, friend, sister, and so on. Penn and Frankfurt (1995) believe these voices are unfinished and therefore capable of being changed and modified through healing conversations with others. Listening to narratives from women in families and communities can move the nurse beyond the tendency to categorize and label according to a so-called normative model, in which all families are considered and measured as if these were universal standards.

Unheard voices and how culture factors serve to quiet voices of minority females in single family households should be regarded as comprehensive care is provided.

Little space has been given to the multiple voices and experiences of working class and minority women in families (Collins, 1991). Since we all grow up under the gaze of the dominant culture, alternative female narratives have been either ignored, stereotyped, or deviant (Weingarten, 1994). As a result of internalized socially constructed expectations, women in families may become silent to their experiences often at great risk for their health.

When factoring class, race, and gender, the nursing literature often fails to include the space in which the poor, black woman-headed household live out their lives. Images of such women are projected and reinforced by the media and the larger community as intergenerationally doomed and overwhelmingly dysfunctional (Collins, 1991). "Behaviors are described as if they can be discussed separately from social, political, and economic contexts" (Bridges & Lyman, 1993, p. 34). Such women fall silent, retreat into the shadows, and become marginalized as their perspectives are not acknowledged. Marginalization condemns your voice to little or no credibility within public discourse. Marginalization grants other people the power to define you, and to remove your autonomy established through self-definition.

Constrained by cultural images of their lives as other voices speak for them, blacks become disconnected from a society that defines women in families so restrictively. Women often feel a profound contradiction between what is actually experienced and what others in the mainstream expect them to experience (Bassuk, 1993).

The nursing literature is beginning to rise to the challenge of including in the dialogic space the patient's worldview as equally useful as the professional's point of view. To the extent that the dominant culture speaks for these women and silences their voices, healthcare delivery becomes irrelevant, "technically correct" but spiritually ineffective (Penn & Frankfurt, 1995).

The case study illustrates how the silencing of a poor African American woman can obstruct enlightened care. Describing Ms. J. in a traditional manner, the nurse would view Ms. J. as a single woman coping ineffectively with the heavy demands of caregiving. She becomes another of "those mothers," invisible to the health workers who have difficulty listening to voices outside of their own personal experiences.

Denigration of single motherhood diverts attention away from the social context in which mothers are forced to go it alone. Single motherhood most often intersects with poor educational achievement, unemployment, low income, and/or abusive relationships. Cultural tales about fathers presume that their absence from the home is the source of most family problems (Weingarten, 1994). The issue of making room for fathers in families is critically important. Weingarten states, "I would rather the public conversation about absent fathers become one about competent, caring fathers and be committed to the kind of work it would take for this to happen" (p. 159). An additional corollary is that in a healthcare system in which all voices are legitimate, the public discourse would also be about being committed to competent, caring communities that are life sustaining for families. Each of these explanations is not competing truths but different perspectives with different implications for how change is to occur (Anderson & Goolishian, 1994).

Unable to organize her experiences in a narrative that gives meaning, possibilities, and a context for change, Ms. J. sought out numerous agencies, looking for solutions to problems she was unable to define in some contextual manner. Caring for herself, her three children, and the growing child inside of her was draining her energy, both physiologically and emotionally. She talked during the interview about being disconnected and lacking in intimate contact. She had a need for connectedness beyond the role of nurturer.

Ms. J. became silent because she believes she has no voice or story to tell. When people feel defective they tend to feel trapped and paralyzed. Often the price paid for such silence is to perpetuate the cycle of poverty into the next generation. She needs to be in conversation in order to understand her experiences in the context of class, race, and gender. The extension of internal conversation to external conversation changes perspective and opens the window for choices in recasting her story (Weingarten, 1994).

The Transformational Nurse and Empowerment

Traditionally, nursing has steered people to adapt to their suffering, rather than to challenge it. The paternalistic professional model is one in which social and personal problems experienced are categorized and defined by the professional through diagnoses. The patient then becomes labeled and the responsibility for a solution is shifted to powerful people who develop treatment plans, and then develop another label, noncompliance, if these plans are not followed. Clients often distrust healthcare workers and view their care as meddling, irrelevant, or inappropriate. Ms. J. reflects this feeling when she told the nurse, "I took my son to be evaluated and he began to play games with him. A week later, I got this report in the mail. I don't believe or understand this report and I still need help, which I am now wondering if I will ever receive."

The failure to connect with Ms. J. and to provide life-sustaining support are based on the underlying societal cultural dynamics that can influence therapeutic relationships with women and particularly African American women (Stevenson & Renard, 1993). "There is still a paucity of information about specific behavioral interactions . . . that will be perceived as credible . . . given social stressors that makes the experiences of African Americans and other oppressed minorities different from majority-culture clients" (p. 433).

The nurse must first recognize and challenge her own preconceived assumptions. Next she must be sensitive to the oppressive issues which can stimulate many emotions of mistrust (Stevenson & Renard, 1994). The caring and empathic nurse must maintain a culturally relativistic perspective; that is, to understand client's behavior within the context of his or her own culture (Martin & Henry, 1989; Outlaw, 1994).

The traditional goal of the helping relationship was to do for people in need rather than to support people to identify and address their own needs. The doing or serving type of help has played a key role in silencing the voices of women in families. Relationships of dominance impede autonomy and making choices because these type of relationships are about control and restricting choices.

The nurse can collaborate with Ms. J. in unlearning cultural messages that restrict her in having control over her body and her life. Health as empowerment is the control of one's life through mobilization of community resources. The community resources include finding powerful metaphors for internal experiences by gaining access to groups as support for validation of experiences. The validation would include confronting distortions, self-criticism and reframing experiences in such a manner that would enable Ms. J. to be more forgiving of and compassionate with herself (Zimmerman & Dickerson, 1994). People cannot change when their behavior is negatively connoted. Empowerment is about feeling at ease in and in charge of one's body and making choices.

A transformational nurse would empower Ms. J. to give voice to her experiences, thereby finding creative space to define her life in a choice-enhancing fashion rather than as a victim. Making meaning out of one's experiences is the beginning of recasting one's story in a different perspective, thereby creating a context for change. Rescripting her life, means that Ms. J. will experience herself differently. She can then take control of her family's destiny, choosing alternatives that have been awakened in her. This liberation can extend into reframing the legacy that she passes on to her children and her community.

As long as Ms. J. believes that she is voiceless, she will feel powerless and trapped by the cultural myths and the lives that went before her. Empowerment allows her to use the creative space that locates self outside the prevailing, ideological claims for victim status, and to rework the story in terms of who she can be.

Last, nurses need to understand the larger social issues of social justice and social policy. Responding to critical human and environmental needs are important, but doing this only in the form of direct service without a parallel concern about the societal policies or cultural habits that create these needs may actually perpetuate the underlying problems and foster further dependence (Bassuk, 1993).

_____ANNOTATED REFERENCES_____

Anderson, H., & Goolishian, H. A. (1992). The client is the expert: A not-knowing approach to therapy. In S. McNmee & K. Gergen (Eds.), *Therapy as social construction* (pp. 25–39). Newbury Park, KS: Sage.

The book presents a concept of therapy as the client's presentation of his worldview and the modification of his perspective in personal dialogue with the therapist and significant others.

Bassuk, E. (1993). Social and economic hardships of homeless and other poor women. *American Journal of Orthopsychiatry, 63*(6), 340–347.

This article compares and contrasts the phenomenon of homeless women to homeless men. Women have the additional burdens of marginalization, parenthood, and the crumbling support of the extended family as poverty, drugs, and other ills take their toll.

Bridges, J., & Lynam, J. M. (1993). Informal carers: A marxist analysis of social, political, and economic forces underpinning the role. *Advance Nursing Science, 15*(3), 33–48.

The authors challenge nurses to develop ways to empower informal carers of elderly adults so that these caretakers will develop alternative choices rather than just coping with the present situation.

Clarke, P. N., & Cody, W. K. (1994). Nursing theory-based practice in the home and the community: The crux of professional nursing education. *Advances in Nursing Science, 17*(2), 41–53.

The authors believe that theory-based nursing practice is hindered by an educational system that educates students in hospital institutions to carry out doctors orders. They discuss why they believe that community-based practice and experiences is where nurses will learn about people, health, and a holistic perspective for independent nursing practice.

Collins, P. H. (1990). *Black feminist thought.* New York: Routledge, Chapman and Hall.

The author explores the experiences of black females inside and outside the academia, examining such areas as work, family, oppression, controlling images and stereotypes, sexual politics and relationships, and finally, the theory of Afrocentric feminist epistemology.

Marable, M. (1995). *Beyond black and white.* New York: Verso.

The author describes how race, as it has been understood within American society, is being rapidly redefined, along with the basic structure of the economy with profound political consequences for all sectors and classes.

Outlaw, F. (1994). A reformulation of the meaning of culture and ethnicity for nurses delivering care. *Medsurg Nursing, 3*(2), 109–111.

The author discusses dimensions of caring necessary to deliver culturally sensitive care that transcends transcultural nursing.

Penn, R., & Frankfurt, F. (1995). From monologue to dialogue. *Family Process, 33,* 220–231.

The authors discuss the concept of "voice" from a social constructionist perspective. They believe that patients enter therapy with narratives or worldviews that are unfinished and self discovery comes about through entering into dialogic space with others, including the therapist.

Stevenson, H. C., & Renard, G. (1993). Trusting ole' wise owls: Therapeutic use of cultural strengths in African-American families. *Professional Psychology: Research and Practice, 24*(4), 433–442.

This article describes the development of cross-racial psychotherapeutic strategies by a white trainee who is being supervised clinically by an African American psychologist.

Weingarten, K. (1994). *The mother's voice.* New York: Harcourt Brace.

Drawing on case histories and personal experiences, the writer, a family therapist and mother of two, discusses the crippling cultural messages about women and motherhood.

West, C. (1993). *Race matters.* Boston: Beacon Press.

The author believes that race is a social and political construct rather than a biological reality.

Zimmerman, J., Dickerson, L., & Victoria C. (1994). Using a narrative metaphor: Implications for theory and clinical practice. *Family Process, 33,* 233–245.

The authors describe a type of family therapy in which there is an emphasis on personal stories that people have created to make meaning out of their experiences.

Chapter 13

BUILDING TRUST

Shirlee Drayton-Hargrove

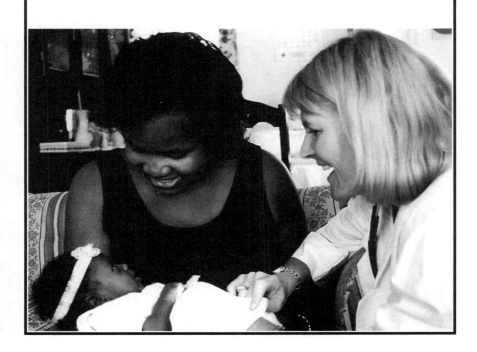

COMMENTARY

Vernice D. Ferguson

In the first case study presented, Dr. Drayton-Hargrove offers five valuable suggestions to reduce conflict and enhance collaboration at the community level when new programs are conceived and implemented. These suggestions become useful first steps in leveling the playing field. Oppressed individuals and populations perceive reality quickly. Being slighted or ignored are everyday occurrences for so many of them. Nurses would do well to note this concern and act on it when plans to work within a given community are considered.

The second case study underscores once again the basic human desire to be treated with respect. Developing sensitivity to clearly communicated messages as well as subtle ones must be ever before us. When we fail to keep this in mind as we do our work, opportunities are lost for improving the health of the public.

Community Partnerships

1. Examine the struggle for trust and acceptance of nursing interventions in community settings.
2. Identify issues of social control that lead to resistance and inhibit cross-cultural communication and collaboration.

*N*urses have formally provided care to individuals in community settings since the work of Lillian Wald in the Henry Street Settlement almost 100 years ago (Barger & Rosenfeld, 1993). However, given the poor health of minorities and low-income groups, the need for nursing centers that provide primary care has been re-evaluated. The goal of community-focused care is to facilitate the biopsychosocial well-being of individuals linked socially, economically, politically, geographically, and historically. As America becomes more ethnically diverse and nurses become increasingly involved in the care of people in their homes and in nursing centers, barriers to cross-cultural collaboration surface.

After reading a local health department report that documented the poor health status of a traditionally underserved community, 6 Anglo-American nursing faculty from a large urban university decided to submit a federal grant for a new community nursing center. The community surrounding the university was 95 percent African American. Most of the families in this community had annual incomes below the poverty level. Families often used the emergency room for primary as well as acute healthcare since many were underinsured and had no access to preventive services. The community health report revealed that the local population had a higher morbidity for HIV/AIDS, tuberculosis, cardiovascular disease, and certain cancers.

The nursing faculty worked diligently over several months studying the literature and documenting the need for a nursing center. Several approaches to community members were made to discuss feasibility of the nursing center. Letters validating its need were written. One faculty member noted that a local church would make a great location for the nursing center since its constituency drew largely from the surrounding community. Before the grant was submitted, a member of the church's board of trustees suggested that the church house could be considered as a potential site. After tremendous work, clear demonstration of need and good intent, the grant was submitted and the nursing center was funded with this church as a tentative site.

The involved faculty members then made an appointment with several church members to discuss plans to open the center in the fall of that year. On the meeting day, the 6 nursing faculty members arrived early and toured the local community. During the meeting, the few community members in attendance and the church trustees had very little to say. The chair of the church trustee board was their spokesperson. The nursing faculty members shared their plans to have a nurse practitioner several days during the week, health fairs, childbirth, and nutrition classes. To the surprise of the nursing faculty, the church trustee chair announced with very little explanation that the church would no longer be available for the nursing center.

QUESTIONS

1. What are the obstacles to the success of this church-based nursing center?
2. Why were there opposing views of the situation?
3. What are the barriers to cross-cultural collaboration?
4. How can a shared culture of understanding be achieved in this situation?

ANALYSIS AND DISCUSSION

What went wrong? Each group created differing stories to explain what went wrong. Each explanation had its own interpretation. The nursing faculty shared their disappointment with the breakdown of "the agreement" within their professional community. "We followed all the procedures," they asserted. None of the nursing faculty could understand why the church community would refuse their "generous" offer to provide healthcare services to a community with so many serious health-related needs. The faculty members expressed concern that the church and community members were "resistant" to the help being offered, and noncommunicative about problems, if they existed at all. "How can we help them if they won't let us?" the nurses lamented.

The church and community members shared their different perceptions of the situation in community circles. They were disturbed to learn about a large grant being awarded to the nursing department that would be totally administered by the university. "Why can't the church be a partner with the university and share the administrative cost?" they said.

The nursing faculty members were viewed as being condescending and self-serving. Many community members expressed resentment about "six Anglo-American persons" coming into "their community" to provide healthcare without even asking what services were wanted or needed. One church member noted, "How would they feel if six African American nurses came into their community church and told them what they needed? Certainly there are some African American nurses these days, they just cannot come in and take over."

Further, the nursing faculty's proposal to provide care for several hours over three days during the week was viewed as insufficient. The grant called for a full-time nurse practitioner. "Why didn't the nurse practitioner work full days and some evening and weekend hours?" some asked.

Although the nursing faculty and community members had communicated throughout the grant-writing process, their views about the nursing center's development diverged. Each group presented differing views of reality. They selected facts to interpret events to fit unexpressed feelings and expectations. Much can be learned from this situation by nurses seeking cross-cultural collaboration with communities. Five points will serve as a guide to facilitate trust and acceptance in community-focused interventions. These points can reduce the conflicts over social control that lead to resistance and inhibit cross-cultural collaboration.

Communities Have a History. A community is often linked by common ethics, values, beliefs, celebrations, and a particular history (Bernal, 1993; Gigler & Davidhisar, 1991; Spector, 1991). Nurses must have knowledge of this history and respect its importance. In this case the community is 95 percent low-income African American, with a history of being oppressed and subordinated. The church serves as a major social center in many African American communities (Dubois, 1986). The church fills the spiritual and psychosocial needs of many. For many African Americans the church may represent the one place where influence and self-actualization is experienced. Therefore, the church often speaks for the community on important issues.

A history of economic underdevelopment, racial bigotry, and oppression has systematically kept African Americans in a subordinate position

(Browning & Woods, 1993; Dubois, 1986; Grier & Cobbs, 1968). This fact cannot be ignored as the nurse interfaces with this community. African American communities confront the reality of epidemiological trauma in their daily lives. African Americans continue to fare more poorly than the general population (DHHS, 1993). The infant mortality rate is double that of whites (DHHS, 1990). African American males have a higher mortality rate than white males (DHHS, 1990). African Americans are more likely to be uninsured and have less access to healthcare, compared to whites. To further complicate the problems, they are more likely to live in poverty.

Many African Americans are cautious and rightly so. In our society there seems to be growing opposition to group rights and a long-standing anti-egalitarian tradition (Omi & Winart, 1983). Distrust is far reaching and is based on a history of disparities in treatment. Immoral experiments such as the Tuskeegee experimental disease project have made people more cautious about what services they will accept from powerful sources. There cannot be an assumption that trust exists in cross-cultural collaboration. Trust must be earned.

Nursing faculty members with decision making and financial power were viewed as (1) condescending, (2) self-serving, and (3) disrespectful. The community members wanted to avoid situations that placed them in the position of being an unequal partner. Being sensitive to the history of a group means that nurses must engage in extensive negotiation and joint planning when developing healthcare services (Jezewski, 1993).

Community-Focused Joint Planning. Community-focused healthcare is not merely based or stationed in a community in a particular location but is defined by the needs of the individuals who comprise the community (Bernal, 1993). How then can nurses design community-focused strategies to facilitate healthy lifestyles without the involvement of people who will be recipients of the interventions?

In this case, church members did not feel involved in the planning of the "nursing center" from the very beginning. They perceived that this center was for nurses and was not really a center for them. They felt excluded from decision making and the ability to define their own needs was marginalized. The power to decide financial matters was exclusively by the nursing department and the university, while community members needed to be increasingly involved in the planning at every step of the project.

The goals of the project must be made clear with emphasis on the community to reduce competitiveness. The community should be oriented to the reasons for the project. The benefits for the faculty and the community should be clearly stated to reduce disorientation and fear. Trust of the nurses is important to develop early in the process. There must be ongoing dialogue and data sharing to reduce barriers of mistrust and cautiousness.

Decision-making processes should be designed to enhance joint participation, interdependence, and outcomes that meet the needs of the persons in the community. The sequence of the project's implementation should be clearly and jointly defined in the planning stages. In the case described, unresolved planning issues such as the schedule of the nurse practitioner facilitated mistrust, competitiveness, conflict, and confusion.

Paternalism, Unequal Power, and Control. Touring the community without leadership from respected and trusted community members should not be done. It is becoming increasingly unacceptable in 1995 for an all-white nursing group to work in a primarily African American community. Culturally-linked faculty members who reflect the makeup of the community should be involved in the planning process. This person or persons should not simply be a "show-piece" but should hold a position of authority in the planning committee. If the person of color is available simply to demonstrate the presence of minorities on the project, this will be viewed as patronizing and dishonest. If an all-white group enters an African American community from a position of control, unequal power, and disrespect, then the alarms will sound in the form of oppositionist stories that reverberate throughout the neighborhood. These stories can be destructive to projects needed by neighborhood people. Nurses must know that control, power, and respect must be shared and are essential to the helping relationship.

Perceived Exploitation of the Needs of the Poor. The nurse and the community should develop collaborative relationships based on mutual trust and respect. In planning community-focused services there must be a win-win situation. Essentially the nurses cannot expect to be the winners of a large federal grant with the ability to purchase computers, new supplies, as well as enjoy the elevated prestige among their peers while the community feels their gains are lesser. In other words, grants cannot be written based on perceived needs of the poor that primarily benefit the advantaged professional. Equality means the community must stand to win the things *they have defined as essential,* for example, the need for evening and weekend services involving, counseling, birthing, and nutrition classes. The key to success means encouraging the community to define the needs of its members, and to share in the jobs created by the grant, an approach based on joint ownership of the project rather than of university/professional control.

Nurses Must Be Knowledgeable of Culture But Sensitivity Is the Key. Mere knowledge of the history, beliefs, values, and traditions of a community does not produce culturally-competent professionals. Sensitivity is the key to such competence, an awareness of the biopsychosocial needs and values of others (Warda, 1995). It involves caring enough about the health of diverse populations to make their needs and values come first. Sensitivity gives healthcare professionals a tool to resist an unconscious tendency toward social control in the form of paternalism and the perpetuation of unequal power relationships. Sensitivity involves the personal validation of history and differing worldviews. Sensitivity involves a respect for the history of the community that will guide the actions the nurse takes on the community's behalf. To be an effective cross-cultural collaborator, many helping professionals must engage in critical self-evaluation. Comfortable and long-held feelings of dominance must be relinquished. This will involve the reconstruction and reordering of values and attitudes concerning human respect and dignity. The outcomes for helping professionals would involve gaining new awareness and increasingly effective skills in cross-cultural collaboration. However, sensitivity is essential to successful multiculturalism (Warda, 1995).

This case examines a situation of mistrust and resistance to social control that inhibits equality and cross-cultural collaboration. Five points were presented to enhance the effectiveness of community-focused care intervention and to enhance the understanding of cultural meaning.

ANNOTATED REFERENCES

Barger, S., & Rosenfeld, P. (1993). Models in community health care: Findings from a national study of community nursing centers. *Nursing and Health Care, 14*(8), 426–431.

This article reports the findings from a national study of community nursing centers. The structure and functions of a plurality of nursing centers providing primary care to traditionally underserved client populations are discussed. The high standard of educational preparation of registered nurses employed at community nursing centers, the reimbursement and income level, and the characteristics of client populations are emphasized.

Bernal, H. (1993). A model for delivering culture-relevant care in the community. *Public Health Nursing, 10*(4), 228–232.

A model of cultural-relevant community practice is presented. In this model, cultural self-awareness, self-efficacy, social supports, and community are key concepts toward the delivery of culturally relevant care in community health agencies.

Browning, M. A., & Woods, J. H. (1993). Cross-cultural family-nurse partnerships. In S. I. Feetham, S. B. Meister, & J. M. Bell (Eds.), *The nursing of families: Theories, research, education, and practice*. Newbury Park, CA: Sage.

This article highlights the development of cross-cultural family-nurse partnerships as a model for nursing interventions. The authors examine the health issues of racially diverse and low income groups. The deteriorating health status of racially and ethnically diverse people with low incomes is reviewed and presented as evidence of the lack of access to health services in those communities. Ethnocentricity and racial guilt are contrasted and examined as a deterrent to the development of cross-cultural nurse-patient partnerships.

DuBois, W. E. B. (1986). *The souls of black folk*. New York: Vintage Books/The Library of America.

This classic book emphasizes the struggles of black American. W. E. B. Dubois highlights the problem of the color line in the twentieth century and the effect of racism on African American life. This book also highlights the cultural pride and resilience of African American people.

Giger, J. N., & Davidhizar, R. E. (1991). *Transcultural nursing: Assessment and intervention*. Philadelphia: Mosby Year Book.

This book presents the components of culturally appropriate care. The authors utilize a guiding framework that focuses on six key cultural phenomena—communication, space, social organization, time, environmental control, and biological variations. The authors proposed that these key concepts provide a model for examining diverse populations.

Grier, W., & Cobb, P. (1968). *Black rage*. New York: Bantam Books.

This book is a classic account of the cruelty of racism. The reverberation and institutionalization of racism is discussed. Grier and Cobb illustrate and explore the rage that has become a part of African American life.

Jezewski, M. A. (1993). Culture brokering as a model for advocacy. *Nursing and Health Care, 14*(2), 78–85.

An advocacy model is presented to serve as a guiding framework to assist patients to overcome barriers in the health care system. The health care system is viewed as a diverse cultural system. The author describes intervening dynamics of patient/provider and power/powerlessness. Stages in the model include the examination of perception, intervention strategies, and outcome evaluation. The author proposes mediating, negotiating, intervening, sensitizing, and innovating as key strategies of the cultural broker.

Omi, M., & Winart, H. (1983). Racism is prevalent today. In B. Leone (Ed.), *Racism: Opposing viewpoints* (pp. 137–143). San Diego, CA: Greenhaven Press.

This article examines the prevalence and realities of racism. The authors examine racial politics, racial restructuring, traditional racist morality, spatial deconcentration, and individualism as racist. The authors predict turbulence in race relations and that race relations will be deeply embedded in the overall crisis of American politics.

United States Department of Health and Human Services. (1990). *Healthy people 2000: National health promotion and disease prevention objectives* (Publication No. PHS-91-50212). Washington, DC: Government Printing Office.

This book profiles the health status of Americans with emphasis on special age groups and at risk populations. The nation's goals to increase the span of healthy life for Americans, to reduce health disparities, and to achieve access to preventative services is presented. The national objectives for health promotion and disease prevention are documented.

United States Department of Health and Human Services. (1993). *Toward equality of well-being: Strategies for improving minority health* (Publication No. ISBN-0-16-04174-7). Washington, DC: Government Printing Office.

This book outlines the long-range goals of Office of Minority Health for the tracking of minority health programs and health status improvements. Goals and objectives for cancer, cardiovascular disease, diabetes, HIV/AIDS, intentional violence, infant mortality, and substance abuse are presented. Goals and objectives related to access and financing of care, data collection, and underrepresentation in the health professions are also addressed.

A Guest Is in My House

OBJECTIVES

---

1. Examine the cultural dynamics that influence therapeutic relationships between nurses and clients in the home setting.
2. Examine barriers to cross-cultural communication in therapeutic interactions.

A new visiting nurse arrived at the home of Mr. and Mrs. Smith for a previously scheduled appointment. It was the first home visit by a nurse since Mr. Smith was discharged from the hospital. Mr. Smith is an 80-year-old African American who needs extensive care due to severe hemiplegia caused by a recent cerebrovascular accident. When the nurse arrived, several ladies in Mr. Smith's room were engaging in prayer. The nurse greeted the individuals whom Mrs. Smith introduced as "sisters" from her church. Mrs. Smith said she felt very tired since her spouse often required care throughout the night. She explained that the church sisters helped care for Mr. Smith by allowing her periods of rest. The nurse instructed Mrs. Smith and the sisters to leave the room so she could perform Mr. Smith's physical assessment in private. After completing the examination the nurse gave Mrs. Smith a list of instructions on how Mr. Smith's care "should be delivered." The instructions included range of motion exercises and bowel and bladder management. Mrs. Smith was instructed to turn her husband more often since he had a beginning decubitus ulcer on his sacrum. During the interactions, Mrs. Smith was referred to as "Alice." After packing her supplies, the nurse said good-bye to Mr. and Mrs. Smith and hurried to her next appointment.

Mrs. Smith was very upset over this home visit. She complained to the local visiting nurses' agency requesting a reassignment of nurses. Later that day, the agency's supervisor called the nurse to share the elements of Mrs. Smith's complaint.

Mrs. Smith had told the supervisor, "The nurse was rude to me and my friends who came to support me in my husband's care. She interrupted our prayer. The nurse ordered my friends and me out of my husband's room. She rushed through my husband's care like a machine. She gave these brief canned instructions and told me what to do and then criticized the care I have been giving my husband."

The visiting nurse was in disbelief after hearing the nature of the complaint. She perceived that she had adequately performed the critical assessment and had given thorough instructions to Mrs. Smith within the time constraints of her workload.

―――――――――――――QUESTIONS―――――――――――――

1. Why was Mrs. Smith upset over the events that transpired in her home?
2. Why did this nurse lack awareness, knowledge, and sensitivity to the cultural meaning of home care?
3. What are the barriers to cross-cultural communication in therapeutic interactions?
4. How can the nurse facilitate cross-cultural communications in therapeutic interactions?

―――――――――ANALYSIS AND DISCUSSION―――――――――

The first encounter in the patient-nurse relationship is critical. The nurse failed to recognize important cultural aspects of family life. She was a guest in Mrs. Smith's home, a place of personal control for the Smith family. Mrs. Smith resented the lack of power, diminished control, and perceived paternalism over the events occurring in her home once the nurse arrived. The nurse was perceived as an authority who sought to regulate the events in the Smith's home and influence how they related to each other.

The "church sisters" were an important part of Mrs. Smith's extended family, a culturally significant communal relationship. They held allegiances to each other and were there to assist in the provision of care to both Smiths and because the nurse was insensitive to the role these individuals played, Mrs. Smith and her church sisters felt excluded from the process of caring for Mr. Smith. Instead, the nurse was perceived as an abusive intruder who had arrived to assume a position of power over the women in their house.

The nurse's communication style prevented her from getting to know the family. She lacked understanding of the interdependent relationships in this family. She relayed cold facts about how Mr. Smith's care should be administered and officious directions with which Mrs. Smith was expected to comply. Although the nurse did not intend her remarks as criticism, Mrs. Smith heard the directions and the instructions on the way care should be provided as a criticism of the care that had been administered to her husband to date.

Mrs. Smith expressed frustration with her husband's care needs, but the nurse ignored her feelings. Emotion is an important cultural aspect of communication in many African American families. By ignoring Mrs. Smith's feelings, the nurse communicated disregard for her emotional needs and expectations. The nurse failed to actively listen. No time was spent clarifying Mrs. Smith's understanding of care requisites. The nurse asked no questions about Mr. Smith's care before she proceeded with her tasks. Praise and encouragement for Mrs. Smith's efforts would have validated her difficulty and emotionally draining work on her husband's behalf.

Spirituality is a critical aspect of African American life (Stevenson & Renard, 1993). Among many African American families, intrusion into prayer ritual is viewed as disrespect for the persons involved as well as their God. During these rituals, all persons are expected to be engaged in the praise of God or be silent. Interruptions should be avoided until the prayer leader concludes the session. Because prayer and spirituality are perceived as critical to well-being and functioning, the nurse's intrusion was viewed as disrespecting an important dimension of the Smith family's life.

The nurse was also accused of rushing through Mr. Smith's care. Nurses, like other health professionals, have time constraints. However, time must be allotted to provide culturally sensitive care (Warda, 1995). In this case, a sociocultural assessment was not performed. Implied in Mrs. Smith's complaint is that the nurse did not care enough about her spouse's well-being to take her time and to be thorough. The nurse failed to sit down and inquire. In the eyes of many African Americans, the needs of people and humankind generally take precedence over time allotments.

Mrs. Smith needed praise, encouragement, involvement, and more explanations concerning her husband's care. She also desired the personal attention of the nurse. Thus, the nurse's systematic rituals and her rushed, mechanistic approach to patient care were deeply resented.

Providing care to patients at home is an intimate experience. Culturally sensitive care requires listening, time "being with," inquiry, and flexibility. Mrs. Smith did not trust the nurse because she violated many of the family's expectations about the establishment of a trusting relationship and rapport with the extended family.

To be more effective, nurses seeking to gain cross-cultural understanding should consider the following challenges and opportunities.

_____CHALLENGES AND OPPORTUNITIES_____

1. *Perform psychosocial and cultural assessments.* Although physical assessment is essential, psychosocial and cultural assessments promote healing by identifying cultural strengths of families and communities (Spector, 1991; Stevenson & Renard, 1993; Warda, 1995). Patterns of interaction are important to identify how group members are interconnected. One of the church sisters may have been the primary care provider and the nurse by failing to take the time to understand such relationships, the nurse in this case may have undermined a potent source of healing power in this family.

2. *Provide respectful care.* Respect is essential in all aspects of health care delivery but it is particularly important when working in communities and the homes of families. Permission must be obtained to move into the personal space of people and to interfere with their rituals. Unfortunately, Western medical practices have given health professionals too much license to intrude into personal environments of people in the guise of operating on their behalf (Spector, 1991).

   In hospital settings nurses typically move in and out of patients' rooms without permission. Nurses should ask for entry privileges even in a hospital setting. The nurse in the case did not request permission to enter the patient's room. Home care must have a family and community focus. The care provided is not simply based in the home but must be comprehensive and focused upon the needs of the individuals, the families, and communities. Respect for privacy, the healing role of prayer and spirituality should be part of nursing practice. Nurse must take time to listen and interact with the patient, immediate family, extended care providers and the community.

3. *Engage in sensitive cross-cultural communications.* Verbal and nonverbal behaviors can foster unwanted dependency, interdependency, or cross-cultural collaboration (Warda, 1995). Simply giving directions, information, and subtle criticisms can cause patients, families, and the community to depend too much on the nurse's leadership rather than their own. Therefore, community-focused care seeks to facilitate leadership in individuals, families, and communities to engage in healthy lifestyles and to cope with disease and illness.

The communication style of the culturally competent nurse respects the feelings of people. Praise and encouragement should be incorporated into care interactions. The ideas of families and community groups should be used whenever possible. The culturally competent practitioners ask questions designed to elicit ideas and problem-solving strategies. The nurse failed to take the time needed to establish rapport, to make a sociocultural assessment, and engage in effective cross-cultural health interactions.

The communication style of the culturally competent practitioner includes formality. The nurse in the case violated the respect that is inherent in calling Mrs. Smith by her surname. In a society in which respect and status is conferred by calling people by their last name or titles, clients should be referenced in a formal manner. Name holds cultural meaning for many people. Therefore, surnames are employed until permission for informal referencing has been granted.

SUMMARY

The nurse's role is to promote patient autonomy, self-determination, and informed decision making (Jezewski, 1993, p. 79). The nurse who seeks to provide culturally-competent care to individuals, families, and communities must perform a sociocultural assessment to determine the repository of strengths and knowledge that these target populations possess (Bernal, 1993; Spector, 1991). Care must be delivered in a manner that demonstrates regard and respect. The verbal and nonverbal communication of the nurse must be sensitive to cultural differences and encourage persons toward actions on their own behalf.

ANNOTATED REFERENCES

Bernal, H. (1993). A model for delivering culture-relevant care in the community. *Public Health Nursing, 10*(4), 228–232.

A model of cultural relevant community practice is presented. In this model, cultural self-awareness, self-efficacy, social supports, and community are key concepts towards the delivery of culturally relevant care.

Jezewski, M. A. (1993). Culture brokering as a model for advocacy. *Nursing and Health Care, 14*(2), 78–85.

An advocacy model is presented to serve as a guiding framework to assist patients to overcome barriers in the healthcare system. The healthcare system is viewed as a diverse cultural system. The author describes intervening dynamic of patient/provider and power/powerlessness. Stages in the model include the examination of perception, intervention strategies, and outcome evaluation. The author proposes mediating, negotiating, intervening, sensitizing, and innovating as key strategies of the cultural broker.

Spector, R. E. (1991). *Cultural diversity in health and illness* (3rd ed.). Norwalk, CT: Appleton & Lange.

This book examines culture, health, and illness with emphasis on provider self-awareness, issues of health of diverse populations, and traditional views of health of diverse populations. Health practices in Asian-American, African American, Hispanic-American, Native-American, and White Ethnic communities are examined.

Stevenson, H. C., & Renard, G. (1993). Trusting ole' wise owls: Therapeutic use of cultural strengths in African-American families. *Professional Psychology: Research and Practice, 24*(4), 433–442.

This article emphasizes the cultural strengths of African American families. The author propose the identification and employment of cultural strengths in families in therapeutic interventions designed to promote health.

Warda, M. R. (1995). Dimensions of culturally competent care. In J. Wang (Ed.), Proceedings of the Second International and interdisciplinary health research symposium: *Health care and culture* (pp. 173–178). West Virginia University School of Nursing, Department of Health Systems.

In this article the author extensively reviews the literature to identify and define the dimensions of culturally competent nursing care. Five central dimensions of culturally competent care are identified: (1) Awareness and sensitivity to cultural diversity, (2) Knowledge of cultural concepts and patterns, (3) Skills in integration of cultural concepts into practice, (4) Focus on interaction of the patients personal cultural variables in an integrated manner, (5) Promotion of an environment in which values, customs, and beliefs are respected.

Chapter 14

THE CHALLENGE OF HIGH-RISK BEHAVIOR

Elizabeth Dickason

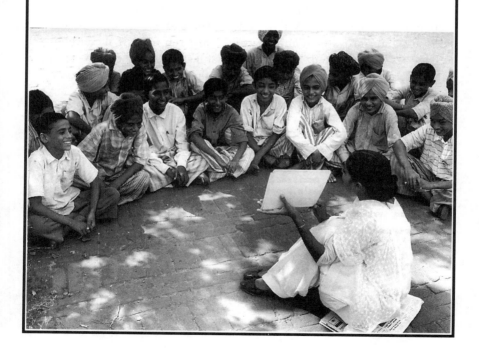

COMMENTARY

Vernice D. Ferguson

Teenage pregnancy and violent behavior are awesome challenges in the United States, exacting high personal and societal tolls. Successful strategies must be directed to the affected teenagers as well as the peer group. In addition, the reach must be extended to the teenager's family and the larger community for a more lasting effect. Identifying helpful opinion shapers in the affected communities is a necessary intervention for success in reducing high-risk behaviors.

Dr. Dickason offers two case studies that are rich for group discussion as creative approaches that are acceptable to those served and have a chance for success emerge. We are reminded that the environment and lifestyle are powerful influences on healthcare outcomes. Teenage pregnancy and adolescent violence thwart countless opportunities for the best life possible for many of today's youth.

Understanding the stages of human development and the impact of race, culture, gender, and class on handling anger and conflict are crucial in making a meaningful impact on the reduction of high-risk behaviors.

Once again, the importance of forming partnerships and mutual planning is recognized. Action plans developed within a given community and across community groups are required if meaningful change is to be effected. Sharing successful strategies should be highlighted, applauded, and replicated when they suit a larger community of interest.

Teenage Pregnancy

————————————OBJECTIVES————————————

1. Analyze and interpret national teenage pregnancy data as it applies to this population.
2. Describe the cultural conflicts in regard to premarital sex and teen pregnancy.
3. Describe appropriate nursing interventions to meet the goal to reduce the number of pregnancies in this population.

*I*n the first 6 weeks of school Ms. S., the school nurse in an inner city high school, has identified eight pregnant freshmen. There are also several additional students who are obviously pregnant, some with their second child. The school nurse would like to develop a program to reduce the number of pregnancies in this population. The demographics of the population include African Americans (55%), Hispanics (40%), and Whites (05%).

————————————QUESTIONS————————————

1. How do the school population statistics for teenage pregnancy compare to national statistics?
2. How do the physical and emotional developmental stages of this population affect the pregnancy rate?
3. How will cultural traditions affect implementation of a program to decrease the pregnancy rate?
4. What strategies would you initiate to change the sexual behavior of these students?
5. What is the impact of your cultural views on the development of a health promotion project to reduce teen pregnancy for this population?

_____ANALYSIS AND DISCUSSION_____

The United States leads the developed world in the number of teenage pregnancies. This has been identified as a public health problem in Healthy People 2000: National Health Promotion and Disease Prevention Objectives. A baseline rate of 71 pregnancies per 1,000 girls ages 15 to 17 was established with a goal of reducing this to 50 pregnancies per 1000 girls (1990). Teenagers represent 24 percent of all births in the United States. Birth rates are highest for African Americans with 186 births per 1000 adolescent girls followed by Hispanics with 159 births per 1000 adolescents (Aretakis, 1996).

The experience of being a teen mother can have a profound impact on the life of the individual. It often means not completing high school, which will impact on the ability of this individual to become self supporting. She may depend on family or governmental assistance in order to provide for her child (Aretakis, 1996). The majority of teen mothers (69%) are not married at the time of the baby's birth and rely on family and social network for support.

Lethbridge (1995) identified some characteristics of the African American culture that influence child bearing. These include a "sex-positive" view of life. Families are more inclined to define their environment by their senses, sight, sound, taste, smell, and touch. People grow up with a great deal of physical affection and this continues through adulthood (p. 459). The extended family of blood relatives and others who provide support is prevalent in the African American community. The view that a baby is the future is dominant in this population. For the adolescent female this may be a strong message that sexual activity and pregnancy are acceptable. In addition, the young African American male may be influenced by peer pressure to engage in sexual intercourse with the expected outcome of a pregnancy. African American males are more apt to father children when pregnancies are common and accepted in their community, and when they perceive fatherhood to be minimally disruptive to their life (p. 460). The preferred methods of birth control in the African American population in hierarchy order are sterilization, hormonal contraception, and barrier methods. While sterilization would not be appropriate for adolescents it may be chosen at a later time following the birth of one or more children.

Among the Hispanic population in the United States are Mexicans, Puerto Ricans, and Cubans. They are often viewed by the dominant culture as one population. Some commonalities shared by the Hispanic population include Spanish language, male-dominated family standard sex roles (Lassiter, 1995).

Cultural norms for the adolescent girl often include an elaborate celebration on her 15th birthday. This event, Fiesta de Quince Anos, signifies that the young female has reached the age for dating and marriage (Lassiter, 1994, p. 55). For the male, the culture belief is Machismo which influences sexual behavior. Machismo relates to the belief in double sex role standards that stresses female virginity and female marital fidelity but encourages male promiscuity before and during marriage. Females are expected to bear the burden of not bringing shame to their families in any manner related to sexual activity, while the males are expected to be openly sexually active which will be accepted in a positive light within the community (Lassiter, 1995, p. 56).

Both populations of teenagers' physical, psychological, and cognitive stage of maturity will be important factors in sexual activity and pregnancy. Physiological maturity is related to early age or menarche which is associated with an earlier age for pregnancy in all adolescents. Teens who experience early menarche initiate sexual active by age 16 and pregnancy by age 18. African American females experience earlier intercourse and pregnancy (Sheaf & Talashek, 1995, p. 35). Psychological maturity is related to weak ego strength which results in sexual acting out and pregnancy. Another factor that contributes to adolescent pregnancy includes low self esteem (p. 36). Cognitive maturity is described as the ability to think and make decisions in regard to reproductive system and its function may preclude taking any action to prevent contraception (p. 37).

Erikson's developmental stage for the adolescent is *identity* versus *nonidentity* which requires tasks that include establishing an identity separate from the family, initiating dating, and a sexual identity. Both of these tasks make a teenage more vulnerable to taking risks that may result in an unplanned pregnancy. Teenagers are often very self conscious during this phase of their development and may not seek health advice from an adult, relying instead on the advice of friends for advice on sexual issues.

The school nurse will have to develop a program that is unique for each population based on the different cultural expectations for sexual behavior. The nurse will also need to be aware of how her own cultural beliefs influence the nursing interventions offered (Russell & Jewell, 1992). Developing an understanding of intercultural communication, which is a process of transmitting and receiving information between two different cultures is an important factor in providing the appropriate nursing care (p. 168). The goal of intercultural communication is to reduce uncertainty and develop trust, which is the key to any successful health promotion project. This process works best in an environmental of sincerity, patience, and a desire to learn.

The school nurse could create this environment by initially holding small classes where trust could be fostered and later adding larger classes.

A strategy that would be beneficial to the success of the program to reduce teenage pregnancy would be to involve the community. For example, the school nurse could invite members of the Parent-Teacher Association to become involved with developing the unique objectives of a program for each group (Russell & Jewell, 1992, p. 165).

ANNOTATED REFERENCES

Aretakis, D. (1996). Teen pregnancy. In M. Stanhope & J. Lancaster (Eds.), *Community health nursing*. St. Louis: Mosby.

The author identifies trends in adolescent births and community nursing interventions that may lead to prevention of adolescent pregnancy.

Lassiter, S. (1995). African Americans. In S. Lassiter (Ed.), *Multicultural clients*. Westport, CT: Greenwood Press.

Lassiter, S. (1995). Cuban Americans. In S. Lassiter (Ed.), *Multicultural clients*. Westport, CT: Greenwood Press.

Lassiter, S. (1995). Mexican Americans. In S. Lassiter (Ed.), *Multicultural clients*. Westport, CT: Greenwood Press.

The cultural diversity of African Americans, Cuban Americans, and Mexican Americans is discussed in separate chapters. The format for each chapter includes communication, family, elderly, child-rearing practices, religious beliefs and practices, cultural dietary practices, morbidity and mortality, as well as beliefs about death and dying. The author presents fifteen separate cultures in a manner that is easy for the reader to cross reference.

Lethridge, D. (1995). Fertility management in Taiwanese and African American. *JOGNN, 24*(5), 459–463.

A discussion of fertility management that includes values and norms of sexual behavior, choice of partners, child-bearing patterns, and the support and resources of the social environment of African American and Taiwanese women.

Russell, K., & Jewell, N. (1992). Cultural impact of health care access: Challenges for improving the health of African-Americans. *Journal of Community Health Nursing, 9*(3), 161–169.

The health status of African American women is described along with an evaluation of the impact of sociocultural beliefs and lifestyle on health promotion, disease prevention, and health maintenance. The authors state that in developing culturally specific nursing intervention the values, beliefs, and standards of the client, health provider, and institution must be included in the plan of care.

U.S. Department of Health and Human Services (USDHHS). (1990). *Public health service. Year 2000 health objectives.* Washington, DC: Government Printing Office.

Healthy People is a national health plan that focuses on disease prevention and health promotion. Specific objectives include: Increasing the life span of healthy Americans, providing access to preventive services to all Americans, and reducing the race-based dispart in life expectancy. Each objective has categories of health promotion, preventive services priorities, and system improvement priorities.

Sheaff, L., & Talashek, M. (1995). Ever pregnant and never-pregnant teens in a temporary housing shelter. *Journal of Community Health Nursing, 12*(1), 33–45.

A cross-sectional study of 136 ever pregnant and never pregnant teens living in a temporary housing shelter. The purpose of the study was to describe differences in selected demographic, sociocultural, physiological, psychological, and cognitive variables in these groups.

Adolescent Violence

1. Analyze the influence of values and culture on adolescent behavior.
2. Apply concepts from the behavioral sciences to the junior high school community.
3. Contrast your own cultural values with those of junior high school students.
4. Describe appropriate nursing interventions (programs) for primary, secondary, and tertiary levels of prevention.

*M*s. D., a junior high school nurse, has noticed an increase in the number of students seeking care for physical abuse (i.e., fighting) with a classmate. She has also observed some students harassing other students in the hallways and cafeteria. She is also aware that the trip to the school and back has become dangerous for many students. The youngsters are often physically assaulted and/or verbally abused by classmates or students from other schools.

Ms. D. has discussed this problem with the other school nurses in her district. While the problem is present in all schools, some schools have higher rates of reported violence. The schools are located in the city; students represent primarily African American and Hispanic populations.

The school nurses have requested the assistance of a community health agency in developing a program to reduce the number of physical and verbal abusive behavior incidents in the school.

QUESTIONS

1. How are your cultural values similar/different from the students in the study?
2. How does the student's physical and developmental stage relate to violence?
3. How do this school's statistics for physical and verbal abuse compare to the national statistics?

172

4. What is the impact of different cultural communication styles on violence?
5. What would you describe as the important components in primary, secondary, and tertiary levels of prevention?
6. What is violent behavior?

ANALYSIS AND DISCUSSION

The first step in the process of gathering information regarding the problem of violence in the school system would be to document the number of students with complaints of physical and/or verbal abuse. After gathering this information, it would be helpful to compare the local statistics to the national statistics.

The U.S. Public Health Service (USPHS) has identified teenage violence as a public health problem in their Health People 2000 National Health Promotion and Disease Prevention Objectives (1990). The USPHS recommendation includes two objectives that are designed to reduce teenage violence. A risk reduction objective which states a goal of reducing by 20 percent the incidence of physical fighting among adolescents, and a service and protection objective that states a goal to increase by 50 percent the proportion of elementary and secondary schools that teach nonviolent conflict resolution.

School nurses are aware that violence is described as nonaccidental acts, interpersonal or intrapersonal, that result in physical or psychological injury to one or more persons. Assault among teenagers often results in long term health conditions such as head injuries, spinal cord injuries, and abdominal stomas from gunshot wounds as well as emotional trauma. Therefore, primary prevention is critical to the well being of the teenage population (Campbell & Langenberger, 1996).

An understanding of the factors associated with violence for this age group will be essential in developing an appropriate program to reduce the number of incidences. There are community factors that contribute to violence within the general population that may be seen. If this occurs it will also be reflected in the teenage population. An additional factor is the influence of television and the movies, which depict physical assault and verbal abuse as ways to handle anger and conflict (Prothrow-Stith & Spivak, 1992).

Erikson has described the interaction of emotional, cultural, and social forces on personality development which leads to the achievement of *ego identity*. *Ego identity* involves accepting oneself and having the skills for healthy functioning in society. The stage of development for the 12- to 18-year-old is described as *identity* versus *identity diffusion*. The purpose of this stage is to develop a sense of self, a set of values and a belief system. Adolescents accomplish this task by trying on various roles, and receiving responses from others. The adolescent who is not able to develop an identity or direction will have *identity diffusion* (Marlow, 1973).

The junior high student is in the early stage of completing the tasks for the identity developmental stage. They are experiencing physical changes which alter their body image, initiating dating, developing friendships with the same and opposite sex, as well as beginning to pull away from their family (Marlow, 1973).

Characteristics of teenagers that increase their propensity for violence include their self consciousness which makes them vulnerable to verbal attacks and often leads to a physical altercation. Peer pressure is a major determinant affecting the behavior of adolescents. As young people separate from families and develop their own identity, the need to belong to a group increases (Prothrow-Stith & Spivak, 1992). If the group believes that physical assault and verbal abuse are the accepted behaviors then the adolescent will conform to these expectations.

In addition to completing the requisite developmental tasks, the African American adolescent has to develop a healthy racial identity. Adolescents may respond to racism with anger which increases the chances for a personal confrontation (Lassiter, 1995).

The cultural influences during this time would be significant to their achieving mastery of this developmental stage. In some instances, the cultural values and beliefs may increase the risk of violence between different groups.

African American culture has a family structure that includes the extended family with strong kinship bonds that is based on shared decision making. The roles of the members are flexible and interchangeable and the degree of authority is linked to the economic provider and not gender (Logan & Semmer, 1996). Kinship bonds and flexibility of family roles are adaptive strengths. The communication style often seen in the African American culture is animated, loud, interpersonal, and confrontational. Some African Americans believe that violence increases when their unique communication style is restricted (Lassiter, 1995). African American English uses words and pronunciations that differ from standard English used in the mainstream culture. African Americans like to be close when communicating. They have direct eye contact when listening and look away when speaking. Also, they do not always use eye cues to indicate whose turn it is to speak. This is opposite to speaking patterns of most Whites (Lassiter, 1992).

In the Hispanic culture, the family structure includes a large extended family as well as close friends identified as family and referred to as "fictive kin." The male in the family is the provider. If he is unable to fulfill this role, he will experience decreased self-esteem and respect of the family. The language that is frequently spoken is Spanish. It is usually spoken rapidly and at a high volume which creates a problem within mainstream society because it may be perceived as hysteria. Many Hispanics believe that it is rude to disagree with an authority figure so they remain silent. However, they may not comply with the directions of the authority figure. They prefer a close personal space in their interaction with others and view touch as an acceptable means of communication (Lassiter, 1992).

Because the communication styles of both cultures may be misinterpreted by others, an important strategy in a primary prevention program for conflict resolution would be to discuss the unique qualities of each communication style. It is also important to remember that all of the students will be self-conscious in initial meetings. Equally important for the Hispanic male is not to diminish his status. The African American students should be encouraged to develop a healthy racial identity during these group meetings.

Further considerations would be to develop a program that would include activities that would allow the authority figure (teacher/nurse) to function as facilitator thus decreasing the problem with the Hispanic students appearing to agree with the health promotion ideas and later disregarding them. The ability of African American males to be flexible would allow them to have multiple roles in the group and could further add to the development of a healthy racial identity.

A secondary level of prevention strategy would focus on developing safe pathways to school. The nurse has identified that many of the assaults have happened on the way to school. The adults residing in the community might provide security by their presence along the streets to school. Homes could be identified as places that teens could go to if they were being confronted by others. Information regarding the influence of violence in the media could be distributed to the community. For example, suggestions for nonviolent television and movies could be developed by the school nurses and the Parent Teachers Association.

Tertiary prevention would speak to meeting the developmental needs of adolescents who have been injured by violent actions. This would include medical care that would allow the individuals to attend school and enhance the chance for successful completion of the *identity* versus *identity diffusion* developmental task.

———————————————ANNOTATED REFERENCES———————————————

Campbell, J., & Landenberger, K. (1996). Violence and human abuse. In M. Stanhope & J. Lancaster (Eds.), *Community health nursing*. St. Louis: Mosby.

The authors examine the influence of social conditions, economic conditions, population density, and community resources on the increasing violence in communities. They look at individuals, families, groups, and others who become abusers and/or victims.

Marlow, D. (1973). The normal pubescent and the normal adolescent: Their growth, development and care. In D. Marlow (Ed.), *Pediatric nursing*. Philadelphia: Saunders.

The normal growth, development tasks, and health problems of adolescents are presented.

Lassiter, S. (1995). African Americans. In S. Lassiter (Ed.), *Multicultural clients*. Westport, CT: Greenwood Press.

Lassiter, S. (1995). Cuban Americans. In S. Lassiter (Ed.), *Multicultural clients*. Westport, CT: Greenwood Press.

Lassiter, S. (1995). Mexican Americans. In S. Lassiter (Ed.), *Multicultural clients*. Westport, CT: Greenwood Press.

The cultural diversity of African Americans, Cuban Americans and Mexican Americans are discussed in separate chapters. The format for each chapter includes communication, family, elderly, child-rearing practices, religious beliefs and practices, cultural dietary practices, morbidity and mortality, as well as beliefs about death and dying. The author presents fifteen separate cultures in a manner that is easy for the reader to cross reference.

Logan, B., & Semmes, C. (1996). Culture and ethnicity. In B. Logan & D. Dawkins (Eds.), *Family—centered nursing in the community*. Menlo Park, CA: Addison-Wesley.

Presents an overview of culture, ethnicity, and health in several families including, Irish, Mexican, African American, and Native Americans. Implications and strategies for community health nurses that enhance nursing effectiveness include avoidance of ethnocentrism and stereotyping.

Prothrow-Stith, D., & Weissman, M. (1991). *Deadly consequences.* New York: HarperCollins.

The authors address the social context in which adolescent violence occurs and offer strategies to reduce violence in communities. A health promotion project initiated by Prothrow-Stith and Spivak to reduce violence in an inner city is presented.

U.S. Department of Health and Human Services (USDHHS). (1990). *Public health service. Year 2000 health objectives.* Washington, DC: Government Printing Office.

Health People 2000 is a national health plan that focuses on disease prevention and health promotion. Specific objectives include increasing the life span of healthy Americans, providing access to preventive services to all Americans, and reducing the race-based disparity in life expectancy. Each objective has categories of health promotion, health protection, preventive service priorities, and system improvement priorities.

Chapter 15

RECONCILING IMMIGRANT VALUES

Jane Brennan

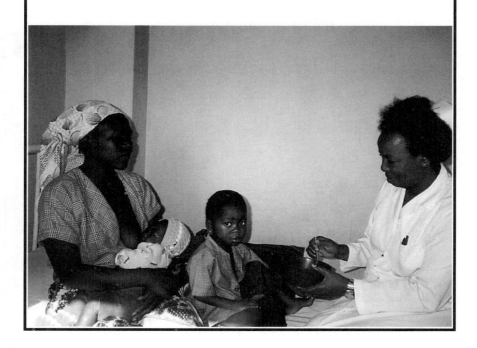

COMMENTARY

Vernice D. Ferguson

Dr. Brennan presents a case study that provides a description of how illness is viewed and treated in another culture. Bringing cultural meaning to what presents itself is of critical importance as assessments are made and assistance offered. The nurse detected an odor of alcohol on the older Jamaican woman, yet noted that she did not appear impaired by alcohol. It is important to know that in Paula J.'s culture rum baths are often used to reduce fever.

The second case presentation helps us to appreciate the impact of the cultural values of a traditional family who has immigrated to the United States. Although ours is a nation of immigrants, we often lose sight of the accommodation that new immigrants must make to the dominant culture as they protect those values that are of importance to them. In addition, conflicts often surface between the generations as young family members struggle to live in two or more cultures, that of their parents and grandparents, the dominant American culture, and that of the peer group with which they identify.

Listening to what people are saying to us and making cultural assessments without judging are tools that nurses must master as they assure acceptable and appropriate care.

A Jamaican Woman

1. Discuss the familial relationship patterns found in the Jamaican culture.
2. Describe how the native Jamaican spiritual and folk healing beliefs and practices influence healthcare.
3. Identify specific communication interventions to facilitate delivery of healthcare to Paula J.
4. Develop a realistic plan of care for Paula J. that integrates her ethnic family and health belief values.

*P*aula J. is a 64-year-old woman who has been experiencing fevers and a persistent cough on and off for the last three weeks. She immigrated to the United States from Jamaica about 20 years ago. A widow, Paula J. lives alone in an apartment near her daughter and son-in-law. She has no primary healthcare provider. Paula J.'s daughter brings her to the Community Nursing Center. The nursing student assigned to the Community Nursing Center observes that Paula J.'s daughter is very solicitous, affectionate, and sympathetic with her mother and seems very anxious about her mother's health. Around her neck, Paula J. is wearing a small, foul-smelling cloth bag. The nurse detects an odor of alcohol but the patient does not seem to be at all impaired by alcohol. When the nursing student takes a nursing history, she finds that Paula J. offers little information about her symptoms.

QUESTIONS

1. What are the predominant ethnic beliefs related to health and illness?
2. How can an understanding of the usual communication patterns among Jamaicans facilitate the nursing student's assessment of Paula J.?
3. Describe some potential communication problems that may arise as a result of language difference.

4. What cultural conflicts between the Jamaican culture and Western medical traditions are important for the nursing student to know?
5. What is the significance of the cloth bag Paula J. is wearing?
6. What is Paula J.'s most likely health problem?
7. How does an understanding of family values figure into the plan of care?
8. List three priority nursing diagnoses and describe the nursing interventions you would use.
9. What cultural remedies are alluded to in the above scenario? (Answer: Use of rum baths for fever, bush teas.)
10. What understanding of the Jamaican community would be helpful to the nurse in providing client care? (Answer: Health beliefs, female-centered culture, extended family responsibility for family members, hospital as last resort, acceptance of male nurses/female physicians.)
11. What spiritual beliefs are common? (Answer: Use of gris-gris, belief in magic.)
12. What effects might language differences have on accurate communication of health-related information? (Answer: Embarrassment on the part of the patient, fear of being perceived as stupid or ignorant.)

ANALYSIS AND DISCUSSION

Communication skills: Ability to express respect and caring through non-verbal as well as verbal interactions.

Assessment skills: Observations, normal lung sounds, heart sounds; knowledge and skill in history taking, physical examination; importance of family history of illness patterns; awareness of significance of variables, such as nutrition, exercise patterns, common childhood illnesses, exposure to infectious diseases; differences between primary, secondary, and tertiary prevention; basic knowledge of how a nursing center provides care.

To be able to provide culturally competent care for Paula J., the nursing student needs to appreciate that illness is both a frequently discussed subject and an anxiety-producing event for most Jamaicans. The psychosocial or spiritual aspects of illness are viewed as more important than the biological aspects. Therefore, Mrs. J. is likely to be experiencing some anxiety about her symptoms. She may blame the illness on sorcery or think of it as a punishment from God. The gris-gris (the foul-smelling bag) is considered to have magical properties.

Recognizing the cultural emphasis on the psychosocial aspects of illness should guide the student to develop a rapport with Mrs. J. through expressions of sincere caring before discussing the signs and symptoms of her problem. From the traditional Western point of view, the nursing student may be tempted to conduct a physical examination initially, suspecting a communicable respiratory disease based on the presenting symptoms. However, this examination should be conducted only after appropriate time has been spent establishing rapport.

Knowing that self-medication is the cultural norm, the nursing student should nonjudgmentally seek information about which folk remedies Mrs. J. has tried. Mrs. J.'s choice of home remedies may shed some light on her perceptions of the particular health problem. The odor of alcohol, without signs of impairment, may suggest the use of rum baths to bring down fevers.

Competency in intercultural communication is a necessary skill, and the nursing student must recognize potential communication barriers. "Healthy intercultural communication begins with an authentic desire to understand someone else's way of seeing the world and acting within it" (Nance, 1995, p. 255). The usual class and language distinction that exists between physicians (who are predominantly male) and average Jamaicans is not likely to be found in the setting of the Community Nursing Clinic, where listening and individualized caring are the accepted values, and women are the primary care providers. Mrs. J. may expect the healthcare provider to tell her, not ask her about her illness. Interpretation of the various clues described above can enable the nurse to meet this expectation.

In planning care for Mrs. J., the nursing student must recognize the strength of the relationship between mother and child which characterizes the Jamaican culture. The greatest personal catastrophe for a Jamaican is the death of one's mother (Wedenoja, 1991). Therefore, Mrs. J.'s daughter may exhibit high levels of anxiety about her mother's condition. Sick persons, whether children or adult, expect attention, sympathy, and nurturance. Family members, especially daughters, expect to be involved in providing care, no matter what the inconvenience (P. J., personal communication, June 20, 1995).

Three priorities of nursing care for Mrs. J. include: accurately assessing her psychosocial and physical status, fostering effective communication, and incorporating both ethnic and traditional approaches in Mrs. J.'s treatment plan. Knowledge of "culture brokering" may be useful in negotiating, mediating, and innovating to achieve congruence between the practitioner's perception of pathology and the patient's perception of illness (Chalandra,

1995). Integration of the family as caregivers will be therapeutic as well as practical.

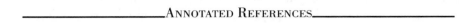

ANNOTATED REFERENCES

Chalandra, M. (1995). Brokerage in multicultural nursing. *International Nursing Review, 42*(1), 19–22.

Culture brokering, defined as mediation between groups with different beliefs and customs, provides a practical framework for nurses working with clients from different cultures. Suggested benefits of this model include a more realistic treatment plan, increased congruence between patient and caregiver, and increased adherence to the treatment plan.

Nance, T. A. (1995). Intercultural communication: Finding common ground. *JOGNN, 24*, 249–255.

Use of a functional perspective toward communication and culture enables clinical practitioners to accept and adapt to differences they encounter in their patients. Goals of intercultural communication include reduction of uncertainty and promotion of trust to create shared meaning.

Seivwright, M. J. (1982). Nurse practitioners in primary health care: The Jamaican experience: Part II. *International Nursing Review, 29*(2), 51–58.

Although somewhat dated, this article illustrates that Jamaican clients highly value kindness, patience, and pleasantness in their healthcare providers, although this is not the pattern in traditional medicine. Clients appreciated the increased availability of primary healthcare made possible through the use of nurse practitioners.

Wedwenoja, W. (1991). Mothering and the practice of "Balm." In C. S. McClain (Ed.), *Women as healers* (pp. 76–97). New Brunswick, NJ: Rutgers University Press.

Through a description of the healing practice of "Balm," the reader gains insight into the health beliefs and practices among Jamaicans, as well as an appreciation of the role of women in Jamaican society.

A Korean American Teenager

_____OBJECTIVES_____

1. Describe the cultural conflicts experienced by Korean American teenagers.
2. Develop at least two alternate plans of care for the individual described in the case study.
3. Propose nursing interventions that are culture specific for the individual.

*L*isa is a 17-year-old high school student in a suburban school district outside a major city with a large Korean American population. Although Lisa and her sister were born in the United States, her parents were both born in Korea and theirs was an "arranged" marriage. Her grandparents come to the United States to visit every three or four years, and she and her parents return to Korea during the interim. Lisa's father is a university professor; her mother is a housewife.

Lisa appears at the high school infirmary one morning wan and teary. She complains of nausea and reports that she has vomited each morning for the past month. Lisa is afebrile and does not appear to be dehydrated. She does not complain of abdominal pain. Lisa has never been to the infirmary before, and the school nurse has never met her. She is aware that Lisa is one of the top students in her class and plans to attend college after graduation. Lisa seems close to hysteria and begs the school nurse to help her.

_____QUESTIONS_____

1. What do you think is the health problem that Lisa is experiencing?
2. How do the traditional Korean family values contribute to Lisa's concerns?
3. What makes Lisa's visit to the school nurse significant?
4. What intercultural communication problems may arise in this situation?

5. What options of healthcare are available to Lisa?
6. Discuss the cultural implications related to each of Lisa's options.
7. Does Lisa's cultural background place her at particular risk?
8. How do the Korean practices related to childbirth relate to this case study?

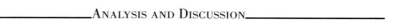

ANALYSIS AND DISCUSSION

Lisa's age and symptoms (morning nausea) suggest the possibility that she may be pregnant. From a cultural perspective, this would be a major tragedy in Lisa's family. The traditional Korean view of sexuality is puritanical, and virginity is highly prized in marriage (Crane, 1972). Pregnancy outside of wedlock would shame not only the individual, making her an "unperson," (Crane, 1972), but also the entire family (Choe, I., personal communication, June 25, 1995; Lee & Cynn, 1991). This cultural value contrasts sharply with the permissive attitude toward sexual activity that prevails in American culture.

To further complicate matters, the prevailing indicator of success among second generation Korean Americans is high academic achievement with pursuit of professional careers at prestigious universities. Lisa's academic performance to this point has reflected this cultural value. An unexpected and unwanted pregnancy creates a major obstacle to achieving the expected success, and thus an added intergenerational cultural conflict.

An understanding of the Korean American culture is essential for the school nurse to effectively communicate with Lisa. Lisa's visit to the school nurse is unusual for her; her high level of anxiety and request for assistance should be seen as indications of a problem of crisis proportions. Awareness that Korean Americans tend not to tolerate secrecy by children and exert strict parental control (Uba, 1994) can further help the school nurse in understanding the complexity of Lisa's dilemma. In interpreting Lisa's communication responses, the nurse must recognize that maintaining an agreeable manner is considered polite and not necessarily a sign of acceptance (Kim, 1995).

In considering potential options of care for Lisa, the school nurse must take into consideration the religious orientation as well as the ethnic background. For example, although many of the cultural traditions of Korean Americans can be traced to Confucianism, many of the Korean American immigrants are Christian. Therefore, an alternative such as abortion might be acceptable based on Confucianism (saving face for the family), but prohibited based on Christian values. Should Lisa be pregnant and desire to have the baby, she is at risk of being exiled from the family. Such a situation would isolate Lisa not only from family support but also from the folklore and traditions associated with childbearing, including food preferences and taboos (Choi, 1986). Should Lisa choose to have the baby, she would need access to prenatal healthcare and delivery services. Little is known about Korean American cultural beliefs about placing children for adoption.

Lisa's predicament and the excruciating cultural conflicts it brings place Lisa at very high risk for depression and suicide. The Korean culture discourages open discussion of feelings and seeking out psychological counseling. For Lisa, who is caught in developmental as well as cultural conflict, individual counseling *without* parental involvement may be the most effective intervention.

Culturally sensitive care for Lisa is a complex and challenging task for the school nurse. Consideration of traditional cultural beliefs must be weighed against individual cultural beliefs and practices. Strategies of culture brokering (Chalandra, 1995) can provide a framework for the school nurse to deliver effective and appropriate nursing care.

ANNOTATED REFERENCES

Callister, L. C. (1995). Cultural meanings of childbirth. *JOGNN, 24,* 327–331.

In all cultures, beliefs and values related to childbirth affect all aspects of social life. Nurses caring for childbearing women need to be aware of the meaning of childbirth and the culture specific coping patterns.

Chalandra, M. (1995). Brokerage in multicultural nursing. *International Nursing Review, 42*(1), 19–22.

Culture brokering, defined as mediation between groups with different beliefs and customs, provides a practical framework for nurses working with clients from different cultures. Suggested benefits of this model include a more realistic treatment plan, increased congruence between patient and caregiver, and increased adherence to the treatment plan.

Choi, E. C. (1986). Unique aspects of Korean-American mothers. *JOGNN, 15,* 394–400.

The findings of this descriptive study of 21 Korean American women reveal that many Korean mothers in the United States continue traditional cultural practices related to conception, taboos, and childrearing. One difference was noted in the tendency of the subjects to bottlefeed rather than breastfeed. The impact of a language barrier is addressed.

Do, H. K. (1988). *Health and belief practices of Korean Americans.* Unpublished doctoral dissertation, Boston University. [CD-ROM] Abstract from: CINAHL. AN 1990112630.

The results of this descriptive study reveal a comprehensive set of beliefs about health and illness that synthesize both oriental and Western concepts. Caregivers need to recognize the importance of the family in making decisions about treatments. Recognition of diversity within cultural groups is emphasized.

Kim, E. (1993). Career choice among second-generation Korean Americans: Reflections of a cultural model of success. *Anthropology and Education Quarterly, 24*(3), 224–248.

This article discusses the value which Korean immigrants place on education as essential to success. This model of success creates a strong community force that may have a negative impact on Korean American students.

Ludman, E. K., Kang, K. J., & Lynn, L. L. (1992). Food beliefs and diets of pregnant Korean American women. *Journal of the American Dietetic Association, 92*, 1519–1520.

This study revealed that traditional dietary beliefs and practices during pregnancy remain evident despite cultural assimilation. Respondents were aware of traditional food taboos, even if they did not observe them.

Kim, M. T. (1995). Cultural influences on depression in Korean Americans. *Journal of Psychosocial Nursing and Mental Health Services, 33*(2), 13–18.

Recent studies have suggested that Korean Americans experience a higher prevalence of depression than other ethnic groups. Healthcare providers must continuously enhance their cultural competence to enhance their clinical effectiveness in dealing with this population.

Lee, J. C., & Cynn, V. E. H. (1991). Issues in counseling 1.5 generation Americans. In C. C. Lee & B. L. Richardson (Eds.), *Multi-cultural issues in counseling: New approaches to diversity.* Alexandria, VA: American Association for Counseling and Development.

Korean Americans who are foreign-born but reared in the United States face unique challenges in adjusting to the demands of two cultures. Health professionals who work with this population need to be aware of the mental health problems associated with these conflicts and devise strategies that include both generations.

Uba, L. (1994). *Asian Americans: Personality patterns, identity and mental health.* New York: Guilford Press.

Chapter 3 provides a comparison of characteristics of various Asian American groups. This information contributes to better understanding of specific cultural groups, including Korean Americans.

Ramer, L. (1992). *Culturally sensitive caregiving and childbearing families.* White Plains, NY: March of Dimes Foundation.

The author presents a perspective on various cultural beliefs related to childbearing. Heathcare providers can identify nursing interventions based on individual beliefs and practices.

Chapter 16

SHARED PERSPECTIVES
Caring for the Elderly

Elizabeth Dickason and Jane Brennan

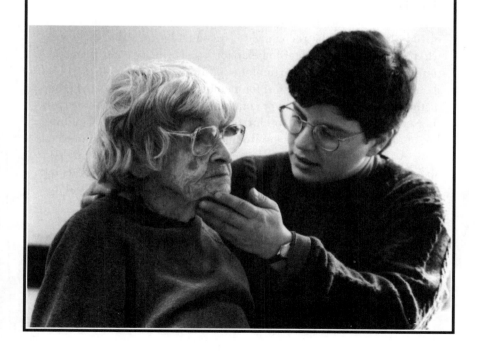

COMMENTARY

Vernice D. Ferguson

The authors of this jointly developed case study are of Irish descent and have been involved in caring for elderly parents. Such a presentation can become a "teachable moment" when presented by members of a particular group. It becomes a vehicle for dialog within and beyond the members of the group described. It opens the door for many points of view including frank disagreement and various shades of agreement and meaning regarding what is a cultural fact or belief. Can the presenting phenomena be labeled as "cultural facts and beliefs"? What is culture? What beliefs and values are commonly shared? Where do environmental factors fit in the transmittal of values and beliefs? What about the individual's educational level, income status, family relationships, the community in which one grew up or lives at present? They become powerful influences on espoused values and beliefs.

Discussion could also focus on labels. Why are they used? Where do they fit? Do they help or hinder understanding? Do labels ever serve a useful purpose? If used how should outliers or exceptions be viewed?

When case studies are used, the need for sensitivity to marginalized groups must be recognized. This must be regarded especially when a socially unacceptable behavior is described rather than a genetic predisposition to a particular condition. Care must be exercised in creating a climate of comfort for members of the marginalized group as the behavior is described or conclusions drawn. This provides further support for the need to clarify definitions, not only of culture, but of race and ethnicity as environmental conditions are factored in.

As Drs. Brennan and Dickason share this case study, many perspectives come into view, not only those of other Irish Americans but those of other cultural groups as well. If nothing more, a mutual and respectful regard for various points of view should emerge.

Caring for an Elderly Parent

1. Assess the health beliefs and practices of a present generation Irish American family.
2. Identify both historical and contemporary perspectives of the family members and potential areas of conflict.
3. Develop a plan of care that includes culturally competent interventions for this family.

*M*ary O'M. is an 87-year-old female of Irish American descent. She has been widowed for 10 years and lives alone in a single family dwelling in a neighborhood that is experiencing socioeconomic change. Mrs. O'M. completed ninth grade, having dropped out of school to care for her 6 younger brothers and sisters when her mother died of breast cancer. She married at 21 and had 6 children in 7 years. Four adult daughters are alive today. One is a lawyer living in Denver, one is an anesthesiologist living in Boston, one is a school teacher in the Philadelphia Catholic School system, and the fourth lives in the same city as her mother. This daughter retired from her position as housekeeper for the parish priests after she experienced a "nervous breakdown."

At Mrs. O'M.'s last physical examination, the nurse practitioner discovered a mass in her right breast about the size of a dime. She underwent a lumpectomy and is currently undergoing follow-up treatment with chemotherapy and radiation. For the past eight years, Mrs. O'M. has been experiencing increasing forgetfulness. Although she was always a fastidious dresser, she no longer appears well groomed. Frequently she will fail to keep an appointment with the hairdresser because, "No one cares about an old lady like me."

Yesterday, the daughter who lives locally received a call from the hospital. Mrs. O'M. had gone out of her house to get the morning paper and was unable to get back in the house. Since it was raining and Mrs. O'M. was dressed

193

only in her nightgown, a new neighbor called the police. Mrs. O'M. was taken to Malaise General Hospital and admitted with a diagnosis of dehydration with changes in mental status. Because Mrs. O'M. was unable to remember her daughters' phone numbers, it was several hours before the family was notified.

The daughters are scheduled to meet with the nurse case manager to resolve the present crisis and to integrate the challenges related to sharing care for their elderly mother.

QUESTIONS

1. Given the cultural background of the family members, what potential conflicts do you anticipate may occur?
2. Discuss three details from the case study which may be explained by culture specific health beliefs and practices.
3. Propose a plan of care which addresses Mrs. O'M.'s physical problems and incorporates the family culture and lifestyle.
4. Who will most likely become the principal caregiver? How will that affect family relationships? Where might feelings of guilt arise?
5. How will the women express their feelings in regard to the change in their relationship with their mother and with each other?
6. How might spiritual beliefs especially those related to sin and guilt affect decisions about end-of-life care?
7. What are some possible physiologic explanations for Mrs. O'M.'s current status?
8. What are the priority issues of care that need to be addressed?

ANALYSIS AND DISCUSSION

- 16 percent of the U.S. population (38.5 million) are of Irish descent.
- Conformity and respectability are highly valued.
- A strong sense of guilt and sin is associated with the Catholic religion.
- Doctors are consulted only in an emergency.
- Some Irish Americans have great difficulty with expressing feelings to close family members.
- Self-control, curiosity, and independence are prized.
- Wearing holy medals is believed to prevent illness.

1. Communication skills with individuals and families.
2. Understanding of family dynamics.
3. Recognition of changes related to aging.
4. Knowledge related to the side effects of chemotherapy and radiation.
5. Awareness of community resources.
6. Consciousness of cultural values and beliefs of Irish Americans.

To be able to provide culturally competent care for this family, the nursing student must be able to assess both physical and psychosocial needs of Mrs. O'M. and her daughters. Mrs. O'M.'s history of assuming responsibility and caring for the family upon the death of her mother may lead her to expect that her children will do the same for her. In planning for Mrs. O'M.'s care, the nurse case manager must be careful not to make assumptions about who may assume responsibility for the mother's care. Careful assessment of family communication patterns will be important in facilitating open discussion and shared problem solving.

An appreciation of the importance of religious beliefs in most Irish American Catholics is needed to help the family examine their choices relating to medical therapy and end-of-life decisions. Mrs. O'M. has many physiological problems which need to be considered along with the impact of normal and pathological changes related to the aging process.

_____Annotated References_____

Martin, C. (1991). Irish Americans. In J. N. Giger & R. E. Davidhizar (Eds.), *Transcultural nursing: Assessment and intervention* (pp. 315–333). New York: Mosby Year Book.

This chapter furnishes information to help healthcare providers better understand the communication patterns and cultural beliefs of persons of Irish American background. Perceptions of space and time and patterns of social organization are also discussed. The chapter concludes with examples of nursing diagnoses, patient outcomes, and nursing interventions.

McGoldrick, M. (1982). Irish Families. In M. McGoldrick, J. K. Pearce, & J. Giordano (Eds.), *Ethnicity and family therapy* (pp. 310–339). New York: Guilford Press.

This chapter offers a paradigm to enhance understanding of the folkways, family patterns, and values of Irish Americans. Although these concepts are presented in the context of a family therapy perspective, nurses and other healthcare professionals can benefit from this knowledge.

Lassiter, S. M. (1995). *Multicultural clients: A professional handbook for health care providers and social workers.* Westport, CT: Greenwood Press.

This handbook offers concise factual information about such topics as communication patterns, family systems and values, socialization patterns, religious beliefs and practices, and culturally based health beliefs and practices. It is useful for healthcare providers in many disciplines.

Chapter 17

A South African Perspective

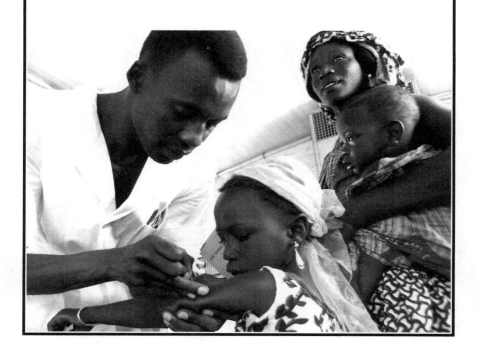

COMMENTARY

Vernice D. Ferguson

South Africa is a multiethnic, multilingual, and multicultural society. Healthcare problems and social welfare concerns embody elements of both the developed and developing world. South Africa is a country experiencing phenomenal political, social, and economic change. At this time of profound change in the healthcare delivery system and its financing, along with welfare reform which is gaining momentum in the United States, it is instructive for us to learn from our colleagues in South Africa.

The case studies that follow serve to remind us of the universality of nursing's work as people are cared for.

Absent Without Permission

Marthie Bezuidenhout

------------------------------OBJECTIVES------------------------------

1. Develop a logical approach to the evaluation of a given situation.
2. Argue the necessity for sound disciplinary policies and procedures.
3. Defend the decisions you would take in handling a given situation.

*T*he key "players" in this case are Mrs. N., the nursing service manager (zonal matron/area supervisor); and professional nurses, June (charge sister), Meg, Grace, and Liz.

Meg had not quite expected what was to happen to her, not two weeks after the incident. Meg was one of four professional nurses working in the dialysis unit. She knew her work was good, she had a good rapport with these patients who were often difficult to handle and had a special knack in canalizing the fistulas. She knew her quality of work was way above that of Grace (a niece of Mrs. N.) and Liz who both requested to work in the dialysis unit because the regular duty hours suited their personal lives and their distance education study program. Meg often wondered why Grace and Liz were placed in this unit because they were both unsuited to deal with and care for this type of patient. They were often impatient and abrupt with patients.

Meg has never objected to working on Saturdays, even though it bothered her that Grace and Liz worked only alternate Saturdays, but then they were younger and possibly received special consideration as they were studying further.

Then the problem arose when Meg desperately wanted to attend the wedding of her best friend in 10 days. She discussed the matter with June, the charge sister, and told her that she thought the obligatory Saturday work was unfair, and that she would in future only work on Saturdays if everyone took turns doing so. Meg stated that she definitely would not work on the day of her friend's wedding. June had agreed to discuss the matter with Mrs. N., but Meg had heard no more about it.

When she returned to work on the Monday after the wedding, June asked her why she had not reported for duty on Saturday. "I attended my friend's wedding," had been Meg's reply.

Two weeks later, Mrs. N. summoned her to the office. What followed was quick and simple. Mrs. N. asked her whether she agreed that she was supposed to work on Saturdays. Meg started to explain that she did not regard this as fair, but was stopped in midsentence by Mrs. N. "Meg, you have worked here for the past two years and, during all that time, you have willingly worked on Saturdays. You cannot now decide that you do not want to work weekends."

Mrs. N. proceeded to interrogate her, firing the following questions at her: Did she admit that she had to work on Saturdays? Had she obtained permission to stay away? Did she admit that she stayed away without permission and without informing anyone? Did she realize this was sufficient reason to dismiss her? Did she have anything to say for herself? Well, if she didn't, that was it. She would have to leave and she would have to agree that management had been fair. She had been given a chance to state her case, but could supply no good reason for her conduct and therefore there was no alternative. She would have to be dismissed.

QUESTIONS

1. Do you think that Meg was fairly treated? Why?
2. Is disciplinary action two weeks after an incident appropriate?
3. Can Meg decide not to work on Saturdays? Explain.
4. Do you think there are ulterior motives for Mrs. N.'s abrupt dismissal of Meg?

ANALYSIS AND DISCUSSION

Meg was not fairly treated. The reason for her termination is insufficient. Besides being substantively unfair, because the penalty does not fit the crime, it is also procedurally unfair (Salamon, 1992, pp. 594–595). Meg did not have the opportunity to state her case and was not given the normal rights of representation, advance notification of charges/allegations, and others under the principles of natural justice (refer to procedural fairness) (Gerber, Nel, & van Dyk, 1995, p. 416; Grossett, 1995, pp. 26–27).

In addition, two weeks had passed since the "transgression" (Grossett, 1995, p. 30). The time limit for initiating disciplinary action is usually no longer than a week, and only where there are unusual circumstances can a delay be justified.

Meg cannot, after two years, decide to stay away on a Saturday. She had accepted the conditions of employment, which probably included Saturday shifts, and even if this was not specifically stated in her contract of employment, she had implicitly accepted it as a condition by not objecting in the past as it was common practice (Sauer & Voelker, 1993, p. 393). She should have insisted that the matter be resolved beforehand and that an answer be given to her question/request about working on Saturdays (Bendix, 1993, p. 258).

One can suspect ulterior motives behind Meg's termination. Mrs. N. brooks no challenge to her authority. There is also a suspicion that Grace and Liz were receiving preferential treatment, and that Meg's departure might create an opportunity for a relative (Bendix & Jacobs, 1991, pp. 238–239, 560).

ANNOTATED REFERENCES

Bendix, S. (1993). *Industrial relations in South Africa* (2nd ed.). Cape Town: Juta.

Sonia Bendix is regarded as an expert on South African labor legislation and the application thereof. This book was written to fulfill a need among industrial relations practitioners and students for a comprehensive reference work in industrial relations, with particular emphasis on the South African situation.

Bendix, S., & Jacobs, F. (1991). *Industrial relations and organisational dynamics.* Cape Town: Juta.

This book fills a real need for experiential and actuality-based learning. It is intended not only for practitioners and trainees in the field of personnel management, but for everyone engaged in the management of people. Typical situations within the work environment are chosen and their correct way of handling is discussed.

Gerber, P. D., Nel, P. S., & Van Dyk, P. S. (1995). *Human resources management* (3rd ed.). Halfway House: Southern.

All three of these authors are academics at the University of South Africa. This book deals with human resources management and all the different facets that affect the employer and employee within the work environment. The development of effective personnel management and application of the current legislation is done in a way that guides the practitioner in his or her day-to-day management of people.

Grossett, M. (1995). *Discipline and dismissal*. Halfway House: Southern.

In this book, the author deals with all the relevant aspects of disciplinary matters and the subsequent procedure if an employee needs to be dismissed. Application of current legislation and procedures within the South African context is explained and clarified.

Piron, J. (1994). *Recognising trade unions*. Halfway House: Southern.

Here the emphasis is on the development and aims of trade unions abroad, and their influence and significance in the South African labor relations scenario. Clarification of the purpose, intentions, and work methods of trade unionism is described and clarified in order for the reader to understand trade unions better.

Salamon, M. (1992). *Industrial relations theory and practice*. New York: Prentice Hall.

This book is intended for students studying industrial relations on undergraduate, postgraduate, or post-experience courses. It provides a framework of knowledge relating to concepts, theories, institutions, and practices of industrial relations in Britain; and to present that knowledge in a way that facilitates the student's learning.

Sauer, R. L., & Voelker, K. E. (1993). *Labor relations structure and process* (2nd ed.). New York: Macmillan.

This book is designed for use in the first course in labor relations or collective bargaining. Although the analysis is relatively sophisticated, it is designed in such a way that no previous background in labor, economics, or business administration is required. This text can be used by students who, either on the management or union side, may become directly involved in labor relations.

Cultural Alienation

Sarie Human

―――――――――――――――OBJECTIVES―――――――――――――――

1. To sensitize students to cultural differences.
2. To make students aware of the implications of culture on healthcare.
3. To create a learning experience for students to analyze a specific case study and to suggest ways of establishing effective, but culturally acceptable healthcare.

*T*he community is a rural village, isolated between mountains. It has a moderate climate with low rainfall, but a consistent river nearby in the grasslands setting. Existing roads, shops, clinics, schools, or other facilities are difficult to access. Transport is by donkey, horse cart, or on foot.

Approximately 100 families live in extended family units. Each family owns several huts which are grouped in a circle and enclosed by a low wall, and known as a *kraal*. All structures are built with a mixture of mud, clay, and cow dung. Outside walls are richly decorated in geometrical patterns in the different colors of clay and mud. The roof consists of conical wooden framework, covered with layers of long thick grass. Each hut has a low entrance used as a door, but no windows. The entrances to huts all face the middle of the *kraal*.

Food, like berries and leaves, is gathered from the veld and crops like maize and sorghum are planted in small pieces of land surrounding each kraal. Fish is caught from the river, and small mammals are hunted by the boys. Cattle are regarded and utilized as a means of payment, and the number of cattle owned by a family is an indication of their wealth. A cow is only slaughtered on exceptional and special occasions, such as weddings and funerals. The cattle are kept overnight in a small enclosed area, just outside of each *kraal*. During the day time, they are allowed to graze the mountain slopes at leisure. The small boys of the families tend to them during the day time. A homemade bell is fitted around the neck of each cow to allow the boys to search for and gather the cattle at night.

Women have a very low status and are not allowed to eat or socialize with the men. The women tend to the fields, gather food from the veld, fetch water from the river, prepare food, build and restore huts, and serve the men. The bigger girls in the families tend to and care for the babies and small children. Men have a very high status in the patriarchal system of the community. Each day they meet with the chief or headman of the village (induna) for meetings (indaba) where the policies of the community are made and discussed. These policies cover all aspects of the organization of the community's daily activities and may include issues such as utilization of land and water, allocation of *kraals*, hearing and disciplining of culprits, initiating children into adult life through rituals and other cultural practices, arranging and agreeing to marriages, etc.

Elderly members are treated with great respect and are cared for by their families. Diseases are mainly treated by the elderly with herbs and plants, and deliveries of babies are done by the old ladies in the communities. Maternal and infant death rates are high. The majority of children suffer from *schistomiasis* (bilharzia) and the incidences of measles in children less than one year of age is the main cause of infant deaths.

At the *indaba* a need for a health service for the community was identified. The community nurse from the nearest primary health care, which is 20 km from the village has been summoned by the men and requested to assist them in building a clinic for their community. They are prepared to provide all the material to build the clinic and also to assist in building it. At the *indaba* a piece of land near the headman's *kraal* was allocated for the clinic and it was decided that one of the headman's daughters could be trained as a nurse to serve the community in the clinic. The community nurse submitted a strong motivation to the local government to build a clinic for the village.

The local government erected a fully-equipped white painted, three-room primary health care clinic, built with bricks, on a piece of land conveniently situated close to the nearest existing road. Services to be offered by the clinic were immunization, antenatal care, deliveries, postnatal care, treatment of common diseases and minor ailments and family planning services. A house for a resident nurse, who would be on call for deliveries during the night time, was erected on the clinic grounds. Arrangements were made with the nearest community hospital (100 km away from the village) to rotate hospital nurses on a two-month basis to the clinic. The hospital used this opportunity to "rid the hospital from the poor and/or the so-called difficult nurses."

The clinic was poorly utilized by the community. The resident nurse was mistrusted by the community. She was lonely and demotivated and wished the three months to pass. No positive change in the morbidity pattern could be illustrated.

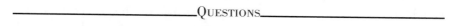

QUESTIONS

1. What are the possible reasons for the clinic being poorly utilized by the community?
2. What are the possible reasons for the mistrust toward the nurse?
3. What approach would you have followed if you were the community nurse who was summoned by the *indaba?*
4. What approach would you have followed if you were the nursing services manager responsible for allocating nurses from the community hospital to the clinic?

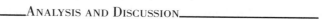

ANALYSIS AND DISCUSSION

Possible reasons for the poor utilization of the clinic include lack of ownership of the clinic by the community. The *indaba* allocated land to the clinic and offered to supply the building material and even assisted with the building of the clinic. This was disregarded. When the *indaba,* which was respected by the community as the highest policy making structure, did not approve of the clinic built by the government, nobody in the community and specifically not the women (because of their submissiveness to the men and their low status) would be allowed, or have the courage to utilize the clinic. It was stated that the existing road was not accessible to the community. The clinic being built close to the road, would therefore have been inaccessible to the community, especially to the sick and to pregnant women. The structure of the building was foreign and could, if it had not been discussed within the community prior to the building of the clinic, result in a culturally unacceptable building.

Strategies toward effective utilization of the clinic include the following: The *indaba* should have received the respect demanded by the community. All decisions should therefore have been discussed and condoned by them. If the land which was allocated by the community was not suitable for a clinic, the reasons should have been explained to the *indaba* and another piece of land should have been negotiated. The community should have been actively involved in the planning, building and implementing of the health services.

Some possible reasons for the nurse feeling mistrusted, lonely, and demotivated include the following: The *indaba* decided that the headman's daughter should be the nurse. Anybody outside their decision would be unacceptable. The criteria used by the hospital for selection of the nurses for the clinics ("nurses who performed substandard and/or being so called 'difficult' and non-compliant nurses"), could result in a negative and prejudiced attitude of the nurse towards the service and the community. The nurse was isolated from her family and/or friends. She had no social support structure in this community and was not accepted and absorbed by the community. She was hospital-oriented and would probably not feel secure and self-confident in a primary healthcare situation. She was also without the professional support structure to consult on professional issues which is available in a hospital situation. The two months which a particular nurse was allocated to the clinic, was not long enough to build a trust relationship and to provide effective and continuous care. No proper community assessment, strategic planning regarding health education and other preventative measures can be planned, implemented, and followed up within two months.

Strategies to address this issue include the following: It should have been explained to the *indaba* that the number of student nurses is limited and that the selection criteria are used with which the headman's daughter would not necessarily comply. It could have been negotiated to appoint the headman's daughter as nursing auxiliary or a volunteer worker or caregiver in the clinic. The nursing service manager should have given nurses, who were interested in gaining experience in a rural primary health clinic, and whose personal circumstances allowed them to leave their homes, the choice of staffing the clinic. Effective orientation, in service training and updating of skills and knowledge regarding primary health care as opposed to hospital care should be offered to these volunteer nurses. The nurse should also be familiarized with the cultural practices and social structures of the community if it is not known to her. The time which a nurse would spend at the clinic would have to be negotiated between the nurse, the hospitals, and the *indaba*. Factors such as time necessary to assess the health needs of the community, long term and short term strategic planning, continuity of care, the importance of building a trust relationship with the community, interest of the nurse in the field of primary health care, acceptability of the nurse to the community, conditions of service contracts, the personal situation of the nurse, and the staffing needs of the hospital, should be taken into consideration. The *indaba* should, if possible, be involved in the final selection of the nurse. Provisions should be made for a professional support system (e.g., two-way radio communication systems, regular and frequent visits to the clinics by competent professional nurses or doctors who are experienced in the delivering of primary health care), a relief system to allow the nurse free time and the opportunity to visit family and friends. A regular top-up system of medicines and other supplies as well as the maintenance of equipment should be provided.

ANNOTATED REFERENCES

Adair, J. (1990). *Understanding motivation.* England: Talbot Adair Press.

Aspects covered in this reference include discussion of motivation and leadership, comparison of motivational models and theories, and application of motivational principles.

Hagemann, G. (1992). *The motivation manual.* England: Gower.

This book covers the field of motivation but also emphasizes the skill and importance of communication, personal development, organizational change, and its implications.

Kinlaw, D. C. (1995). *The practice of empowerment making the most of human competence,* Aldershot, Hampshire, England.

Lazarus, J. (1991). *The process of community-based health personnel development programmes: An international perspective.* South Africa: University of the Western Cape.

An international perspective of community-based health personnel development programmes with a South African perspective.

Stattford, C. S. (1994). *Behaviour at work.* Australia: Cambridge University Press.

Covering aspects such as groups and group behavior, communication, leadership, and motivation.

Understanding and Interpreting Cultural Beliefs

Helga Kirstein

—————————————OBJECTIVES—————————————

1. Identify important characteristics expected from a nurse dealing with other cultures, such as assertiveness, compassion, tolerance, and sensitivity.
2. Recognize the value of being well-informed regarding the cultural beliefs that you encounter.

*I*n South Africa we have a health train that travels to remote rural areas where it then provides different services such as an eye-, dental-, and primary healthcare clinic. The healthcare clinic is manned by nursing staff. At one such location, a 17-year-old Xhosa girl, Loveness Xhumalo, was admitted to the primary health care clinic complaining of hearing voices in her head. Two weeks prior to her visit, Loveness complained of an earache and her aunt who was living nearby, put medication in her ear. This seemed to help for the pain but after a week she started hearing voices in her head.

My general observations revealed the following: Loveness was a tall, slender, and well-groomed girl who, apart from a nervous twitch of her head, appeared to be in good health. She seemed shy and nervous. A general physical examination had to be done carefully as Loveness was obviously not accustomed to being examined by a white female "doctor" as she insisted on calling me. When I wanted to examine her ears, I let her hold the otoscope and she switched the light on while I demonstrated to her how it was used. In her left ear was a tiny beetle stuck in what seemed to be a thick creamy substance. Every time the bug moved, Loveness heard voices and twitched. The utter relief when she realized that it was the bug that caused the voices in her head, was quite rewarding.

1. What medication was put in her ear and why did the aunt do it?
2. Why was Loveness so shy about her condition?

————————————ANALYSIS AND DISCUSSION————————————

The thick cream in her ear turned out to be the fat of a freshly slaughtered chicken that her aunt put in the sun to melt before pouring it into Loveness' ear. Loveness was slow to admit that this aunt was not a relative, but the local traditional healer *(igquira)*. The chicken fat had to be melted in the sun and not over direct heat because it is believed that the strength that lies in the fat would be lost through direct heat. The tiny beetle must have been attracted by the smell of the fat in Loveness' ear.

In South Africa with its many different cultures and religions, the traditional healer plays an important role in the healthcare of many people. A black Christian, for example, may maintain a dualistic approach to illness where he or she adheres to Christian practices and then carries out traditional rites in secret. The more westernized a black is, the more secretive he becomes concerning visits to the traditional healer (Hammond-Tooke, 1989, pp. 103–107). It will take some diplomatic coaching before a client will admit that he or she has been to a traditional healer. In Loveness' case, this was the reason for her initial shyness. She left school when she was 15-years-old and is therefore literate and educated enough to be secretive about her visit to the traditional healer.

A nurse who is exposed to different cultures should realize her limitations in that it is impossible to know everything about every culture that she comes into contact with. Van Tonder (1996, p. 203) states that the nurse should be sensitive and flexible in her professional approach and exercise caution in her assumptions of a given situation.

————————————REFERENCES————————————

Andrews, M. M., & Boyle, J. S. (1995). *Transcultural concepts in nursing care* (2nd ed.). Philadelphia: Lippincott.

Galanti, G. (1991). *Caring for patients from different cultures. Case studies from American hospitals.* Philadelphia: University of Pennsylvania Press.

Hammond-Tooke, D. (1989). *Rituals and medicines. Indigenous healing in South Africa.* Johannesburg: Donker.

Pera, S. A., & Van Tonder, S. (1996). *Ethics in nursing practice.* Cape Town: Juta.

Family-Centered Care

Trinette Derkina Swanepoel

---OBJECTIVES---

1. Study a family as a whole, taking into account that a family consists of individual members.
2. Identify the health needs and health problems of Maria and her family.
3. Describe the roles and nursing interventions a community health nurse does perform in caring for Maria and her family.

*T*his case study involves an African family who are residents of an informal housing settlement. The main theme is culture versus reproductive health and family health needs, addressed by the community health nurse.

Maria is a 24-year-old woman, who suffers from schizophrenia. Her condition is controlled by medication. She receives her psychiatric treatment on an outpatient basis from the psychiatric department at the local hospital. Maria visits the primary healthcare clinic in her area regularly. Here she attends the family planning clinic, where she gets her contraceptive treatment. Maria is the mother of two children. Both children were born by caesarian section and the doctor advised Maria not to become pregnant again. At her last visit to the clinic, the community health nurse noticed that Maria's personal hygiene was unsatisfactory. She appeared depressed, but was well oriented in terms of time and place. During the clinical health assessment, it was found that Maria has sores in her mouth and suffers from halitosis. She also had an offensive-smelling vaginal discharge. Maria is put on treatment. Connie, the community health nurse of that area, decides to pay Maria a visit at home. Connie is concerned about Maria's appearance and evasive behavior.

Maria and her family are living in an informal housing area 20 km from the nearest town. The area is very densely populated. There are no official streets or pavements. Essential provisions are sold at stalls. The permanent primary healthcare clinic in the area is well attended by the members of the community. The hospital is situated in the nearest town. Public transport, in the form of taxis, is available to the nearest town.

Maria and her husband are staying with their two children in a three-room house. The house is built of wood covered by sheets of galvanized iron. The toilet is situated outside in the backyard. The house and toilet are kept clean and tidy. Near the house is a big tree but there is no existing garden. The immediate area around the house is swept clean. Piped water is available 200 meters from the house.

Maria's husband John is home when Connie pays Maria a visit. He is 30 years of age and stays at home because he is recently unemployed. The only source of income for the family is a disability pension that Maria receives. John tells Connie that he is very upset about the fact that Maria attends the family planning clinic. He wants another child. He explains to Connie that it is his cultural belief to have many children.

Children are a man's pride and an indication of wealth. Large families have traditionally been desirable because the children are responsible for the care of their elderly parents. He blames Maria for using contraceptives without his consent. Maria appears depressed when John raises his voice. She then mentions to Connie that John becomes very aggressive at times and sometimes assaults her. John has a very good relationship with his family. His extended family lives close by. Maria states he frequently complains to them that his wife is incapable of having more children. Maria on the other hand gets no support from her family. Maria has a few friends. Maria and John's children are David and Anna. David is five years of age, and his physical and psychological development stages are within the normal limits for his age. He is well nourished, but his hygienic condition is unsatisfactory. His program of immunization is completed according to schedule. Anna is two years old. Her development is somewhat slow for her age. She sits and crawls very well and stands without help, but can walk only with help. She is also well nourished, but her hygienic condition can improve. Her program of immunization is up to date.

―――――――――――――――QUESTIONS―――――――――――――――

1. What are the health needs and health problems of this family?
2. What objectives could be set that will help Maria and her family to satisfy their health needs and solve their health problems?
3. What role does Connie perform in caring for Maria and her family?

4. Who are the members of the multidisciplinary health team that could be involved solving the health problems of this family?
5. What community resources are needed to support this family?

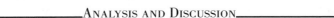

ANALYSIS AND DISCUSSION

Maria and her family are known as a nuclear family, consisting of a mother, a father, and a couple of children. They are staying in a small house, and their only source of income is Maria's disability pension. Although the father suffers no health problems, he is recently unemployed. He gets very aggressive at times and sometimes assaults his wife. Maria suffers from a chronic mental illness, and her current health problems include halitosis, sores in her mouth, and an offensive vaginal discharge.

Connie sits down with Maria and John and listens to their problems. She tries to create a trust relationship. She offers opportunities to Maria and John to air their feelings. As the community health nurse of that area, Connie is conversant with the traditional customs and beliefs of the people of that community. She respects John's view on a large family, but identifies that John is lacking the knowledge of Maria's chronic mental illness and the implications of bearing him another child. Connie asks John and Maria to join hands in seeking solutions to their health problems and promotion of their health needs. Connie explains that she has to perform a family assessment, and that together they should plan the necessary health interventions (Clark, 1992, Appendix F, G, J). John asks Connie to help him to find a job. Connie invites John to visit her at the primary healthcare clinic, and he makes an appointment to see her. Connie plans to help John to understand Maria's mental illness and to counsel him on her health problems. She offers John an opportunity to become part of the "peace garden" community project. She will introduce John to the community leader who organizes the project. Connie initiated the vegetable garden project with money that was donated to her for that purpose. The peace garden is located on the premises of the primary healthcare clinic. Schoolchildren, parents, housewives, elderly people, and unemployed members of the community all participate in the planting, watering, harvesting, and selling of the vegetables. They built their own stall and they market their products to the local people and to the people of the nearby town. The profit that is made is used to develop other community projects in an attempt to create more job opportunities.

Connie makes use of the steps of the nursing process to organize thought processes for clinical decision making and problem solving.

The health needs were assessed (see Table 17–1). Connie looked at the physical-, psychological-, and socioeconomic environment of the family.

Table 17–1
THE FAMILY'S HEALTH NEEDS

Family Members	Physical Environment	Psychological Environment	Socioeconomic Environment
Adults	Safe environment	Love	Financial security
Maria	Proper housing	Affection	Employment
John	Nonviolent neighborhood	Self-actualization	Family interaction
		Self-esteem	Social acceptance
	Basic sanitation	Mental health	Support from friends and family
	Clean water supply	Mechanisms to cope with stressors	Leisure
	Family consumption pattern		
	Basic hygiene	Empowerment	
	Protection against disease (control of medication)		
Children	Exercise	Love	Family interaction
David	Environment free of hazards	Bonding	Opportunities to play with other children
Anna	Playground	Security	
	Proper shelter against heat and cold	Cognitive stimulation	
	Adequate nutrition		
	Basic hygiene		
	Special protection against disease (immunization)		

Connie identified and recorded several health problems (see Table 17–2).

With the input of John and Maria, they set the following objectives:

1. To refer Maria back to the psychiatric department on Thursday for an evaluation on her mental state and to review her medication.
2. To get John involved in the peace garden project as soon as possible.
3. To refer Anna to the medical practitioner at the primary healthcare clinic on Wednesday for a developmental evaluation.
4. To refer John to the social worker at the primary healthcare clinic on the same day that he comes to visit Connie. The social worker may help John to find a job.
5. To help Maria to improve personal hygiene. Maria will attend the health education sessions held at the primary healthcare clinic, together with the children.

Table 17–2
HEALTH PROBLEMS

Family Members	Physical Problems	Psychological Problems	Socioeconomic Problems
Maria	Halitosis Sores in mouth Offensive vaginal discharge Assaulted by husband at times	Chronic mental illness (Schizophrenia) Depression	Low socioeconomic status Disability pension Lack of family support
John		Aggression about his wife's incapability of bearing him more children Conflict with his cultural beliefs	Unemployment Insufficient financial resource Low socioeconomic status
Anna	Slow development for age		
Anna & David	Unsatisfactory personal hygiene		

6. To get David and Anna to socialize with other children. Maria is advised to take the children to a playgroup for preschool children that is held at the church hall on a Wednesday morning from 10:00–12:00.
7. To revisit the family until the health problems are solved and Maria and John are capable of caring for themselves.

Connie performs the following roles in caring for Maria and her family:

Roles	Nursing Action
Clinical	Assessment of the family's health needs (including individual health assessments) Identification of potential and existing health problems
	Early diagnosis, treatment, and care
	Decision making and problem solving
	Protection against disease (immunization)
	Specific health education in connection with health problems identified
	Referral to other members of the multidisciplinary health team
	Home visits and follow-up care
	Practicing community health nursing
Educator	*Health promotion through health education:*
	Maria: Attending of health education sessions at the primary healthcare clinic (e.g., on principles of hygiene, motherhood, good nutrition). Methods used are videos, songs, talks, role play, and group discussions.
	David and Anna: Attending health education sessions for children, involving songs, role play, and puppet shows
	Counselling:
	Maria and John on parenting
	John on his problems

(continued)

Roles	Nursing Action
Administrator (Manager)	Leader of the multidisciplinary health team
	Co-ordinating of the necessary health services
	Facilitating multisectoral collaboration
	Initiating community projects
	Planning of family healthcare
	Organizing nursing interventions
	Record keeping
Advocate	Client advocacy: Explaining to John Maria's mental state and physical condition

To satisfy the family's health needs and solve their health problems, the following members of the multidisciplinary health team should be involved: Community health nurse, medical practitioner, psychiatric nurse, social worker, community leaders, and the minister of religion.

The following community resources are available and accessible to Maria and her family: Primary healthcare services, Department of Welfare, minister of religion, playgroup for preschool children, the peace garden project, family, friends, and neighbors.

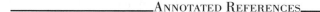

ANNOTATED REFERENCES

African National Congress. (1994). *The reconstruction and development programme*. Johannesburg: Umanyo.

This document comprehends the Reconstruction and Development Programme (RDP), which is an integrated, coherent socioeconomic policy framework compiled by the African National Congress (ANC).

Clark, M. J. (1992). *Nursing in the community*. Norwalk: Appleton & Lange.

This book is designed to provide the nurse generalist with a thorough introduction to all the aspects of community health nursing, to be able to function in any setting where community health nurses practice.

Dennill, K., King, L., Lock, M., & Swanepoel, T. (1995). *Aspects of primary health care*. Midrand: Southern.

This book is the second volume in the series on community healthcare in Southern Africa and provides valuable information for members of the health team working in the field of primary healthcare.

Dreyer, M. (Ed.), Hattingh, S., & Lock, M. (1993). *Fundamental aspects of community health nursing.* Midrand: Southern.

This book is the first in a series of books aimed specifically at the South African community health nurse, and contains an invaluable introductory text.

Edelman, C. L., & Mandle, C. L. (1994). *Health promotion throughout the lifespan.* St. Louis: Mosby.

The focus of this book is on the current trend to emphasize the developing health of the individual, the family, and the community.

Goosen, M. (Ed.), & Klugman, B. (1996). *The South African women's health book.* Cape Town: Oxford University Press.

This book deals with all the issues South African women identified as urgent and important which affect their health, and contributes to the vibrancy of the African women's health movement.

Le Roux, J. (Ed.). (1994). *The black child in crisis: A socio-educational perspective* (Vol. 2). Pretoria: Van Schaik.

This book contributes toward improvement of the black child's situation, more specifically in South Africa, and provide guidelines for the facilitation of positive change.

Stanhope, M., & Lancaster, J. (1996). *Community health nursing: Promoting health of aggregates, families, and individuals* (4th ed.). St. Louis: Mosby.

The unifying theme for this book is the integration of health promotion and disease prevention into the multifaceted role of the community health nurse.

Swanepoel, H. (1992). *Community development: Putting plans in action* (2nd ed.). Kenwyn: Juta.

This book is a plea for participative development, and strives to bring inside to those involved in order to help them to better negotiate the obstacle-strewn path of ground-level development in South Africa.

Theron, F. (1990). *Contraception: Theory and practice.* Pretoria: Academica.

This book contains information on all aspects of reproductive health and strives to contribute to combatting ignorance and prejudice concerning contraception in the South African context.

Van Rensburg, H. C. J., Pretorius, E., & Fourie, A. (1992). *Health care in South Africa.* Pretoria: Academia.

The focus of this book is on the development and structure of the healthcare system of South Africa.

Schizophrenia: The Title Fits Care as Well

Dirk van der Wal

OBJECTIVES

1. To identify cultural congruent demands made by patients and their next of kin within their rights, lack of cultural accommodation and integration by student nurses, educational shortcomings, and unrealistic expectations of teaching a cultural and transcultural component of the nursing curriculum, and possible medico-legal and ethical implications of cultural incongruent care.
2. To discuss these issues and propose alternative solutions to these problems.
3. To recognize cultural stumbling blocks in nursing care and in education.

*T*he case takes place in a psychiatric ward in a Western-oriented medical facility in a rural area. The patient is a traditional African man diagnosed as a schizophrenic with auditory hallucinations. The patient experienced an auditory hallucination: "*Woza, . . . woza . . . Woza kithi. Zibulale! Woza!* (Come . . . come . . . Come to us. Kill yourself! Come!) Mother, who is talking to me." The following exchange occurred:

MOTHER: No one. I do not hear anybody. Hush, come, . . . come . . . quiet now.
PATIENT: Mother, there is a voice telling me to kill myself.
MOTHER: Come, come, there is no one here. There is no one speaking. I do not hear anyone.
PATIENT: It is the spirits of my great grandfathers, the warriors who roamed the plains of Africa. They are calling me to them, to the great plains of lush bush and huge herds of game. They are calling me to the everlasting hunting fields, Mama.

MOTHER: Oh, no! Nurse! Nurse! I must see the *inyanga* [traditional healer]. Now!

NURSE: Sorry. This is a modern medical hospital. We do not have *inyangas* here, only psychologists and psychiatrists.

MOTHER: But you do not understand, the ancestral spirits want to take my son away. We must have offended them. Please, only the inyanga can rid my child from this spell. Only he can satisfy the angry spirits. You must help me! Please, bring the inyanga to us!

NURSE: Come, come. There are no ancestral spirits here! They diagnosed your son as a schizophrenic. It is a mental disease. He believes he hears voices. But, it is only his imagination. There is nothing that the *inyanga* can do! We will treat him with the medicine available, the ones prescribed by the doctor.

MOTHER: Nonsense! What do these doctors know about my ancestors? I do not trust them and I do not believe in them. No, we must take Mkize to the *inyanga* before the spirits become even more agitated. If we do not do so, the spirits will become angry with the rest of his family. He will die. There will be no son for him to honor his name!

NURSE: But, *Mama* . . .

MOTHER: No but's! Are you not a child of Africa yourself? Is it not the spirits of your late great grandparents that watch over you every day? Do you not obey the calls of your ancestors?

NURSE: It is true. Yes, I do obey the calls from my ancestors. Naturally I do. I am a child of Africa. But here I am a nurse and I do as they teach me. If I do not do that they will penalize me. I will not pass my final exams. Here, Mkize is a patient with schizophrenia and we treat him for that.

MOTHER: The spirits are going to be very angry with you. I'll have no part in your sacrilege! I'll take my son to the *inyanga.* I shall!

A clinical nurse tutor who overheard this conversation calls nurse Ntuli to her office.

Tutor: Nurse Ntuli, how on earth do you live with yourself? How is it possible that after everything they have taught you during the past four years that you still believe in ancestral spirits? What utter nonsense! What do you do with your life outside the hospital? How do you set an example for other people in the community regarding mental health? What is your problem?

_____QUESTIONS_____

1. Indeed, what is nurse Ntuli's problem?
2. Did the nurse tutor react appropriately? How should she have reacted?
3. What are the educational problems and implications reflected by this situation?
4. What are the nurse tutor's perceptions of education?
5. How should the student nurse have handled this situation?
6. Are the mother's demands within her rights?
7. How should the student promote mental health in the community?

Skin color is definitely not an issue in this scenario. Please do not read this into the scenario. Do not succumb to the fallacy that cultural differences and lack of cultural competence are always and only attributable to racism. All the characters, including the nurse tutor and the doctors, may well be indigenous black Africans who have undergone a cultural transformation and are quite happy with it.

_____ANALYSIS AND DISCUSSION_____

We encounter several problems in this scenario. Culture issues coming to mind are: cultural alienation, cultural intolerance, cultural island, cultural blindness, cultural conflict, possible indoctrination, wrong expectations regarding teaching cultural aspects, and a number of ethical questions and potential medical legal risks. All of these issues are in some or other way *cultural stumbling blocks* (Andrews & Boyle, 1995, p. 37).

The Mother and Her Demands

Mkize's mother acts culturally within her right to demand that an *inyanga* be brought to her son. Since this is a rural area with a modern Western-oriented medical facility, one would expect for this to be common practice. However, with the nurse's protest to summoning a *inyanga,* the determination of the mother to take her son to an *inyanga* creates a potential medical legal risk. Should the mother really take her son from the hospital premises, and should something happen to the patient, who would be accountable? Can the mother really be held accountable if she acts according to her heartfelt convictions? Having the mother sign a RHT (refuse hospital treatment) form would seem an easy way out of this situation. However, can we really claim, despite whatever information we provide to the mother, that the mother, within her cultural orientation and conviction, her understanding of her son's ailment and her lack of understanding of Western medical diagnoses, can genuinely make an informed decision to sign such a form? We doubt that.

The best solution is to avoid the situation by rendering *culturally congruent care*—incorporate traditional healers into the multidisciplinary team. This implies that nurse Ntuli, and the whole medical facility for that matter, should work more closely with traditional healers. The reassurance that these healers bring to those who believe in their supernatural power is in itself therapy. The traditional healer could also play an active part in promoting the patient's compliance to modern Western medical treatment. The influence these traditional healers have on the everyday living of traditional people should not be underestimated or depreciated. However, presently the health facility can genuinely be called a *cultural island*—an isolated cultural group totally different, and as yet incompatible with the surrounding (dominant) cultural group. Taking into consideration the importance of such a health facility to the people in the community, a policy of reciprocal giving and taking should be adopted.

The Problem of Promoting Mental Health

The question of how nurse Ntuli should, or should not, promote mental health in the community is closely related to the previous problems. Mental health is partly defined by the individual's acceptance of prevailing cultural norms, values, and mores, integrated with personal convictions to form an integrated whole reflecting social acceptance, cooperation, and conformity. If nurse Ntuli could get the cooperation of all the traditional healers in the area and also refer patients to these healers, patients would not be put in the awkward position of having to hear that what they believe in does not exist, or even worse, that it is detrimental to their mental status. Nurse Ntuli would probably do much better if, as a nurse from a *foreign* health institution, she could still convey the message of authenticity to the community by showing that she still believes in and honors the beliefs of her own people.

Nurse Ntuli could spread the word informally in the community that the cooperation of traditional healers would be welcomed, respected, and honored. The traditional networking that exists in traditional communities would soon enough carry the message to those it is intended for. However, more formal communications such as those established between government, traditional leaders, and traditional healers could also be followed.

Nurse Ntuli's Problem

Another serious problem is nurse Ntuli's apparent dichotomous cultural stance. The question here indeed is, *What is her problem?* Her problem is both cultural alienation and poor socialization, and in a certain sense, *culture conflict*. More pertinently, it is a problem of *cultural accommodation*— a process and outcome not yet achieved by nurse Ntuli. This is a problem that no formal education can remedy.

Nurse Ntuli is also experiencing a conflict of interest. We think that this conflict can also be called *cultural conflict* because nurse Ntuli feels threatened by this situation in which she finds herself. She admits to upholding her traditional convictions "out there," however, "in here" she subjects to a very different set of cultural rules, norms, and mores.

Nurse Ntuli needs experience in accommodating different cultural viewpoints and bridging cultural gaps. The experiences needed by nurse Ntuli are definitely not of the formal educational and theoretical kind that border on indoctrination. What nurse Ntuli needs are situations and experiences like the one described, provided they are consummated in an experiential learning format in which instance the nurse tutor should be present to guide nurse Ntuli through these experiences, allowing her to reflect on them. In the situation described, experiential learning, especially reflecting on the experience, is of vital importance to nurse Ntuli's professional development— allowing her to grow.

Conflicting issues need to be clarified with the students and solutions need to be found for any such apparent contradiction and conflicting situations. From an educational point of view, the dilemma nurse Ntuli finds herself in should be anticipated, not avoided. However, anticipated with timely educational guidance in a humanistic and educative caring manner. For instance, value clarification sessions as part of reflection on the situation during experiential learning could be beneficial to students in the clinical field. Naturally, it is not only the nurse tutor that could guide students in this venture. All clinical personnel, staff nurses, ward sisters, and clinical specialists should be involved in this.

The Nurse Tutor's Problem

The nurse tutor's problem seems, to some extent, more serious than that of nurse Ntuli. After all, it can be argued that her possible lack of cultural knowledge, her *cultural blindness*, her tendency toward *stereotyping*, and her apparent unrealistic expectations of, and questionable intentions with, education and teaching could contribute to nurses developing *cultural in-authenticity* (or *cultural marginality* if you wish).

One suspects that her motive with teaching cultural aspects is to convert students, if not bluntly indoctrinating them toward her cultural orientation—unscrupulously promoting *acculturation.* Although a degree of acculturation is perhaps inevitable, it is definitely questionable whether one should pertinently strive to attain a total *cultural conversion* in people. The utmost one could aim for is cultural accommodation and personal low conflict integration of different cultural patterns by any individual—a situation the individual is happy with within a group.

The nurse tutor further seems to be guilty of cultural blindness, by ignoring differences and proceeding as if these do not exist. Many reasons can account for this state of affairs such as cultural intolerance, lack of exposure to cultures other than her own, and consequently, lack of knowledge.

It would be easiest to transfer this nurse tutor, however, in doing so we do not solve the problem but transfer it to someone else to attend to later on. What is applicable to nurse Ntuli is also applicable to the nurse tutor. She needs the necessary exposure to simulated situations, group discussions, role play sessions, values clarification sessions, and clinical experiential learning experiences to guide her toward understanding cultural differences and eventually to cultural tolerance and culturally congruent care.

How Should the Tutor Have Reacted?

The answer to this question is actually given in the discussion above. The nurse tutor should have changed this potentially harmful situation regarding interpersonal relationships, professional integrity and authenticity, and potential medico-legal, ethical, and moral pitfalls into a learning experience. Naturally, changing this single situation into a learning experience would not work wonders immediately for nurse Ntuli, however, a series of such exposures, even in simulated form, might benefit nurse Ntuli.

Acting this way would not only benefit the nurse, but also the patient and his next of kin as well as the institution as a whole and the profession at large. This definitely would have built bridges instead of destroying them.

———————————ANNOTATED REFERENCES———————————

Andrews, M., & Boyle, J. S. (1995). *Transcultural concepts in nursing care* (2nd ed.). Philadelphia: Lippencott.

As a good general source on transcultural concepts, this book contains two chapters on "Transcultural Concepts in Mental Health" and "Religious Beliefs and Nursing Practice" which could serve as background study.

Berglund, A. I. (1976). *Zulu thought-patterns and symbolism.* Claremont: David Philip.

Although an older publication, this source is especially valuable since it deals with its topic of interest from a culturally pure perspective, uncontaminated by westernization and the erosive effect this has on indigenous African culture.

Fairchild, H. P. (Ed.). (1977). *Dictionary of sociology and related sciences.* New York: Littlefield.

This dictionary gives succinct definitions of terms relating to the case study. However, any other social sciences dictionary or a dictionary for anthropology can also be used.

Kavanagh, K. H., & Kennedy, P. H. (1992). *Promoting cultural diversity: Strategies for health care professionals.* New York: SAGE.

This source contains, in addition to a number of case studies, a section on cultural relativism in health which might be of particular interest to students.

Concluding Statement

*I*n nursing, we have come to recognize that there is value in using the case method to enhance learning in new and unchartered practice sites. I was heartened by a comment from a physician educator who asked me about my work with the faculty consortium's initiative in developing case studies. At the time of this query, the two of us were engaged in considerable dialogue with physicians and medical students about multiculturalism as plans for the future were being developed. The physician expressed considerable interest in our initiative and commented, "You nurses are so far ahead of us. The case study ought to be used more often for it appears to be an effective approach to get away from so much didactic instruction. I am interested in your work."

Another interaction comes readily to mind. It occurred early in the 1980s when I served as the nursing leader in what is now the Department of Veterans Affairs. Those of us in the policymaking and executive leadership group became keenly aware of the rapid graying of America, with the veteran population aging 10 to 15 years ahead of the general population. During that period, I took a sabbatical leave and served as Scholar-in-Residence at the School of Nursing, The Catholic University of America. I was able to use the university and its teaching nursing home as a base. I observed care patterns there and in other nursing homes in selected public and private settings from urban to rural America. There could not have been a better way in such a brief time frame to become more aware and informed about long-term care, especially its impact on elders and their care needs. It was a useful way to prepare for the leadership required and policies needed to guide the nursing service as responsive programs emerged based on new knowledge about gerontology and geriatric care.

Concluding Statement

Once again, a physician's comment comes to mind. This time it was a surgeon who expressed no interest in learning specific to caring for aging veterans. He said, "Who needs this training? If a 75-year-old veteran requires an appendectomy, I'll do it just as I perform them on younger veterans? What difference does it make how old he is?"

Score another point for nurses as we strive continually to recognize the need for updating our knowledge in recognition of the dramatic societal changes that are occurring.

In the spirit of change and our need for responding to the public whom we are privileged to serve in an informed and relevant manner, may these case studies in cultural diversity serve you well.

Vernice Ferguson, RN, MA, FAAN, FRCN

REFERENCES

Adams, M. (1992). *Promoting diversity in college classrooms.* New York: Jossey-Bass.

Albrecht, K. (1987). *The creative corporation.* Homewood, IL: Dow Jones-Irwin.

Allen, C. E. (1993, September). Families in poverty. *Nursing Clinics of North America, 29*(3), 377–393.

Allport, G. (1954). *The nature of prejudice.* Garden City, NJ: Doubleday.

Anderson, H. (1992). Hospitals seed new ways to integrate health care. *Hospitals, 66*(7), 26–36.

Anderson, J. (1990). Health care across cultures. *Nursing Outlook, 38*(3), 136–139.

American Academy of Nursing. (1995a). *Diversity, marginalization and culturally competent health care: Issues in knowledge development.* Washington, DC: Author.

American Academy of Nursing. (1995b). *Promoting cultural competence in and through nursing education.* Washington, DC: Author.

American Association of Colleges of Nursing (AACN). (1986). *Essentials of college and university education for professional nursing* (final report). Washington, DC: Author.

American Nurses Association. (1991). *Position statement on cultural diversity in nursing practice.* Washington, DC: Author.

Andrews, M. (1992). Cultural perspective on nursing in the 21st century. *Journal of Professional Nursing, 8*(1), 7–15.

Ardell, D., & Newman, A. (1977, May/June). Health promotion: Strategies for planning. *Health Values: Achieving High-Level Wellness, 1*(3), 100–107.

Bandman, E., & Bandman, B. (1988). *Critical thinking in nursing.* Norwalk, CT: Appleton and Lange.

Beer, M., Eisenstat, R., & Spector, B. (1990, November/December). Why change programs don't produce change. *Harvard Business Review,* 158–166.

References

Beyond the Melting Pot. (1990, April 9). *Time*, 28–31.

Blanchard, F., Lilly, T., & Vaughn, L. (1991, March). Reducing the expression of racial prejudice. *American Psychological Society*, 101–105.

Boyle, J., & Andrews, M. (1995). *Transcultural concepts in nursing care.* Glenview, IL: Scott, Foresman.

Branch, M., & Paxton, P. (Eds.). (1976). *Providing safe nursing care for ethnic people of color.* New York: Appleton-Century-Crofts.

Brink, P. (1987). Cultural aspects of sexuality. *Holistic Nursing Practice, 1*(4), 12–20.

Brink, P. (1989). *Transcultural nursing: A book of readings.* Prospect Heights, IL: Waveland Press.

Burg, M. (1994). Health problems of sheltered homeless women and their dependent children. *Health and Social Work, 19*(2).

Byerly, E. L. (1977). Cultural components in the baccalaureate nursing curriculum: Philosophy, goals and successes. In *Cultural dimensions in the baccalaureate nursing curriculum* (pp. 74–84). New York: National League of Nursing Press.

Capers, C. (1991). Nurses and lay African Americans' views about behavior. *Western Journal of Nursing Research, 13*(1), 123–135.

Capers, C. (1992). Teaching cultural context: A nursing education imperative. *Holistic Nursing Practice, 6*(3), 19–28.

Chrisman, N. (1990). *Expanding nursing practice with culture sensitive care: A new approach to transcultural nursing.* Paper presented at the 1990 Transcultural Nursing Society meeting, Seattle, WA.

Chrisman, N. (1991). Cultural systems. In S. Baird, R. McCorkle, & M. Grant (Eds.), *Career nursing: A comprehensive textbook* (pp. 45–53).

Clark, M. (1995, May/June). Biomedicine, meet ethnomedicine. *Healthcare Forum Journal*, 20–29.

Cox, T. (1991, May). The multicultural organization. *The Executive*, 34–47.

Dailey, M. A. (1992). Developing case studies. *Nurse Educator, 17*(3), 8–11.

Davidhizar, R., & Frank, B. (1992). Understanding the physical and psychosocial stressors of the child who is homeless. *Pediatric Nursing, 18*(6), 559–562.

Davis, B. (1990). Diversity and complexity in the classroom: Considerations of race, ethnicity, and gender. In B. G. Davis (Ed.), *Tools for teaching.* San Francisco: Jossey-Bass.

Davis, G. A., & Scott, J. A. (1971). *Training creative thinking.* New York: Holt.

Davis, L., & Proctor, E. (1989). *Race, gender and class.* Englewood Cliffs, NJ: Prentice-Hall.

Dean, T. (1989). Multicultural classrooms, monocultural teachers. *College Composition and Communication*, (40), 23–37.

Desmond, A. (1994). Adolescent pregnancy in the United States: Not a minority issue. *Health Care for Women International, 15*, 325–332.

References

Division of Nursing, Bureau of Health Professions, Health Resources and Services Administration, DHHS. (1994, February). *The registered nurse population, 1992.* Washington, DC: U.S. Government Printing Office.

Dixon, E., & Park, R. (1990, November/December). Do patients understand written health information? *Nursing Outlook, 38*(6), 278–281.

Elliot, E. (1984, August). My name is Mrs. Simon. *Ladies Home Journal,* 18–19, 150.

Eng, E., Salmon, M., & Mullan, F. (1992). Community empowerment: The cultural base for primary health care. *Family and Community Health, 15*(1), 1–12.

Ethnic diversity: Are we ready for tomorrow's patients and professionals? (1993, May). *Hospitals.*

Farson, R. (1969, September 6). How could anything that feels so bad be good? *Saturday Review of Literature,* 20–21.

Ferguson, V. (1994a, April/May). Challenge and change for a new tomorrow. *Imprint, 41*(3), 57–58.

Ferguson, V. (1994b). The future of nursing. In O. Strickland & D. Fishman (Eds.), *Nursing issues in the 1990s* (pp. 3–21). Albany, NY: Delmar.

Fisher, R. (1990). *The social psychology of intergroup and interactive conflict resolution.* New York: Springer-Verlag.

Fitzsimons, V., & Kelley, M. (1996). *The culture of learning: Access, retention, and mobility of minority students in nursing.* New York: National League for Nursing Press.

Ford, C. (1994). *We can all get along.* New York: Dell Books.

Francis, P. (1991). A review of the multicultural literature. In J. Q. Adams, J. F. Niss, & C. Suarez (Eds.), *Multicultural education: A rationale for development and implementation.* Macomb: Western Illinois University Foundation.

Franklin, J. (1969). *From slavery to freedom. A history of Negro Americans.* New York: Vintage House.

Fuszard, B. (1989). *Innovative teaching strategies in nursing.* Rockville, MD: Aspen.

Galanti, G. A. (1991). *Caring for patients from different cultures. Case studies from American hospitals.* Philadelphia: University of Pennsylvania Press.

Garver, E. (1986). Cultural thinking them and us. A response to Arnold Aaron's critical thinking and baccalaureate curriculum. *Liberal Education, 72,* 245–252.

Geissler, E. (1991). *Transcultural nursing and nursing diagnosis.*

Giger, J., & Davidhizar, R. (1991). *Transcultural nursing: Assessment and intervention.* St. Louis: Mosby Year Book.

Goodwin, N. (1990, October). Health and the African American community. *Crisis, 97*(8), 12, 50.

Hale, R., et al. (1991). Cultural insensitivity in sexist language toward me. *Journal of Social Psychology, 130*(5), 697–698.

Hall, J., & Weaver, B. (1974). *Nursing of families in crisis.* Philadelphia: Lippincott.

References

Hardy, K. (1989). A theoretical myth of sameness: Actual issue in family therapy training and treatment. In G. Sabia, B. Karrer, & K. Hardy (Eds.), *Minorities and family therapy* (pp. 17–33). New York: Haworth Press.

Health manpower requirements for the achievement of health for all by the year 2000 through primary care. (1985). Report of a WHO expert committee (Tech. Rep. Series 717). Geneva: World Health Organization.

Helman, C. (1990). *Culture, health and illness: An introduction for health professionals.* London: Wright.

Hoang, G., & Erickson, R. (1982, August 13). Guideline for providing medical care to Southeast Asian refugees. *Journal of the American Medical Association, 248*(6), 710–714.

Hodgson, A. M. (1972). Structuring learning in social settings—some notes on work in progress. *Programmed Learning Education Technology, 9*(3), 79.

Horton, R. (1967). African traditional thought and Western science. *Africa,* (37), 50–60.

Hufford, D. (1990, June). Culturally sensitive delivery of health care and human services. In S. Staub (Ed.), *Proceedings of the government plenary session: 11. Governor's conference on ethnicity* (pp. 35–37). Hershey, PA: Heritage Affairs Commission.

Johnston, W., & Packer, A. (1987). *Workforce 2000.* Indianapolis, IN: Hudson Institute.

Kavanaugh, K., & Kennedy, P. (1992). *Promoting cultural diversity: Strategies for health care professionals.* Newbury Park, CA: Sage.

Kehrer, B., & Burroughs, H. (1994). *More minorities in health.* Menlo Park, CA: Henry J. Kaiser Family Foundation.

Kleinman, A. (1977). Cultural construction of clinical reality: Comparison of doctor-patient interactions in Taiwan. In A. Kleinman, P. Kunstadter, E. Alexander, & J. Gal (Eds.), *Culture and healing in Asian societies: Anthropological and cross-cultural medical studies.* Cambridge, MA: Schenkman.

Kleinman, A., Eisenberg, L., & Good, B. (1978). Culture, illness and care. Clinical lessons from anthropologic and cross-cultural research. *Annals of Internal Medicine, 88,* 251–258.

Koop, C. E. (1996, Fall). Manage with care. *Time, 148*(14), 69.

Kritek, P. (1994). *Negotiating at an uneven table: Developing moral courage in resolving our conflicts.* San Francisco: Jossey-Bass.

La Fargue, J. (1985, October). Mediating between two views of illness. *Topics in Clinical Nursing, 7*(3), 70–77.

Lechky, O. (1992, June). Health care system must adapt to meet needs of multicultural society, MDs say. *Canadian Medical Association Journal, 146*(12), 2210.

Leininger, M. (1978). *Transcultural nursing: Concepts, theories and practices.* New York: Wiley.

References

Leininger, M. (1981). Transcultural nursing: Its progress and its future. *Nursing Outlook, 11*(7), 365–371.

Leininger, M. (1988). Leininger's theory of nursing: Cultural care diversity and universality. *Nursing Science Quarterly, 1*(4), 152–160.

Levenstein, A. (1976). Effective change requires change agent. *Hospitals, 50*, 71–74.

Lieu, T. A., Nervachek, R. W., & McManus, M. A. (1993). Race, ethnicity and access to ambulatory care among U.S. adolescents. *American Journal of Public Health, 83*, 960–965.

Lipson, J. (1988). The cultural perspective in nursing education. *Practicing Anthropology, 10*(2), 4–5.

Lipson, J., Dibble, S., & Minarik, P. (Eds.). (1996). *Culture and nursing care: A pocket guide.* San Francisco: University of San Francisco Press.

Lipson, J., & Meleis, A. (1985). Culturally appropriate care: The case of immigrants. *Topics in Clinical Nursing, 7*(3), 48–56.

Litman, T. (1975). The family as a basic unit in health care relationships. In *Health of the family: National Council for International Health Symposium* (pp. 159–172). Washington, DC: National Council for International Health.

Locke, D. (1992). *Increasing multicultural understanding.* Newbury Park, CA: Sage.

Mahlangu-Ngcobo, M. (1995). *100 ways of empowering women.* Baltimore: Gateway Press.

Malek, C. (1986). A model for teaching critical thinking. *Nurse Educator, 11*(6), 20–23.

McKinlay, J. (1973). Social networks, lay consultation and help-seeking behavior. *Social Forces,* (51), 273–285.

Meleis, A., Hall, J., & Stevens, P. (1994). Scholarly caring in doctoral nursing education: Promoting diversity and collaborative mentorship. *Image: Journal of Nursing Scholarship, 26*, 177–180.

Meleis, A., Isenberg, M., Koerner, J., Lacey, B., & Stern, P. (1995). *Diversity, marginalization, and culturally competent health care issues in knowledge development.* Washington, DC: American Academy of Nursing.

Miller, M., & Malcolm, N. (1990). Critical thinking in the nursing curriculum. *Nursing and Health Care, 11*(2), 67–73.

Molina, C., Zambrana, R., & Aguirre-Molina, M. (1994). In C. W. Molina & M. Aguirre-Molina (Eds.), *Latino health in the US: A growing challenge* (pp. 23–43). Washington, DC: American Public Health Association.

Nielsen, B., McMillan, S., & Diaz, E. (1992). Instruments that measure beliefs about cancer from a cultural perspective. *Cancer Nursing, 15*(2), 109–115.

Nursing among diverse cultures. (1996, Fourth Quarter). *Reflections, 22*(4).

Orque, M. (1983). Orque's ethnic/cultural system: A framework for ethnic nursing. In M. Orque & B. Bloch (Eds.), *Ethnic nursing care: A multicultural approach* (pp. 5–48). St. Louis, MO: Mosby.

References

Outlaw, F. (1994, April). A reformulation of the meaning of culture and ethnicity for nurses delivering care. *MedSurg Nursing, 2*(3), 108–111.

Overfield, T. (1985). *Biologic variation in health and illness.* Menlo Park, CA: Addison-Wesley.

Putting Gender on the Agenda: A guide to participating in U.N. World Conferences. (1995). New York: The United Nations Development Fund for Women.

Ravitch, D. (1990, Summer). Multiculturalism. *American Scholar,* 337–354.

Ray, M. (1989). Transcultural caring: Political and economic visions. *Journal of Transcultural Nursing, 1*(1), 17–21.

Rinehart, N. (1991). *Client or patient? Power and related concepts in health care.* St. Louis, MO: Ishiyaku Euro America.

Sabatino, F. (1991). Foundations' funding priorities shift from acute to primary care. *Hospitals, 65*(11), 34, 36–37.

Schotfeldt, R. (1978, May). The professional doctorate: Rationale and characteristics. *Nursing Outlook, 26*(309), 302–311.

Schwartz, R., & Sullivan, D. (1993). Managing diversity in hospitals. *Health Care Management Review, 18*(2), 51–56.

Simons-Morton, D. G., Simons, B. G.. Parcel, G. S., et al. (1988). Influencing personal and environmental conditions to community health: A multi-level intervention model. *Family Community Health, 11*(2), 25–35.

Speraw, S. (1987). Adolescents' perceptions of pregnancy: A cross cultural perspective. *Western Journal of Nursing Research, 9*(2), 180–197.

Spradley, B. W. (1991). Cultural dimensions. In *Readings in community health nursing* (4th ed., pp. 51–60). Philadelphia: Lippincott.

Stevens, P., Hall, J., & Meleis, A. (1992). Narratives as a basis for culturally relevant holistic care: Ethnicity and everyday experience of women clerical workers. *Holisitic Nursing Practice, 6*(3), 49–58.

Steward, E. C. (1972). *American cultural patterns.* La Grange Park, IL: Intercultural Network.

Stice, J. E. (Ed.). (1987). *Developing critical thinking and problem solving abilities.* San Francisco: Jossey-Bass.

Strickland, O., & Fishman, D. (Eds.). (1994). *Nursing issues in the 1990s.* Albany, NY: Delmar.

Tappen, R. (1983). *Nursing and leadership: Concepts and practices.* Philadelphia: Davis.

Thomas, E. (Ed.). (1995). *Race and ethnicity in America: Meeting the challenge in the 21st century.* Washington, DC: Taylor & Francis.

Thomas, R. (1991). *Beyond race and gender.* New York: American Management Association.

Tien-Hyatt, J. (1987, May). Keying in on the unique care needs of Asian clients. *Nursing Outlook, 8*(5), 269–271.

Toffler, A. (1974). *Learning for tomorrow. The role of the future in education.* New York: Random House.

References

Torres, S. (Ed.). (1996). *Hispanic voices*. New York: National League for Nursing Press.

Tripp-Reimer, T. (1984). Research in cultural diversity: Directions for future research. *Western Journal of Nursing Research, 6*(2), 253–254.

Tripp-Reimer, T., & Fox, S. (1990). Beyond the concept of culture. In J. C. McCloskey & H. K. Grace (Eds.), *Current issues in nursing* (pp. 542–546). St Louis, MO: Mosby Books.

Valente, S. (1989). Overcoming cultural barriers. *California Nurse, 85*(8), 4–5.

Villaruel, A. (1995). Mexican-American cultural meaning, expressions, self-care, and dependent care actions associated with pain. *Research in Nursing and Health, 18,* 427–436.

Villaruel, A., & Porter, C. (1993). Nursing research with African American and Hispanic people. *Nursing Outlook, 41*(2), 59–67.

Waxler, N. (1974). Culture and mental illness: A social labeling perspective. *Social Focus,* (51), 275–285.

Wheeler, C., & Chinn, P. (1991). *Peace and power. A handbook of feminist pieces* (3rd ed.). New York: National League for Nursing Press.

Yoder, P. S. (Ed.). (1982). *Issues in the study of ethnomedical systems in Africa: African health and healing systems.* Los Angeles: Crossroads Press.

Young-Mason, J. (1997). *The patient's voice: Experiences of illness.* Philadelphia: Davis.

Zweigenhaft, R., & Domhoff, G. W. (1991). *Blacks in the white establishment? A study of race and class in America.* New Haven, CT: Yale University Press.